THE LOST DECADE

HOW HEALTH MISINFORMATION IS COSTING BLACK COMMUNITIES A DECADE OF LIFE

DR. CARLA T. STANLEY

Printed in the United States of America.

For more information or to book a workshop, training, retreat, or event, contact :

ctstanley@comcast.net
https://vitalpathconsultingandeducation.com/

Book design by Honeylette Pino
Cover design by Tri Widyatmaka

ISBN Hardcover: 979-8-9947667-0-5
ISBN Paperback: 979-8-9947667-1-2
ISBN Kindle: 979-8-9947667-2-9

First Edition: June 2026

DEDICATION

For my family, and for every Black family navigating
a system that was never designed for them.

CONTENTS

INTRODUCTION

A Lost Decade

Mary is my aunt.

And on paper, she is not supposed to be the person this book is about.

When people talk about poor health outcomes in Black communities, they often point to familiar factors: lack of education, unstable housing, limited access to care, food insecurity, or growing up without consistent advocacy. Those factors matter. They explain a lot of what we see.

But Mary did not come from that story.

She grew up in a stable, two-parent household in Hammond, Indiana. Her parents were married for fifty years. Her father worked in the steel mills for thirty years. He could not read, but he worked, provided, and showed up. Her mother, Mrs. Thomas, worked part-time in their school cafeteria. The expectation was that children living in this household went to college. Structure and expectation were normal in her life.

Mary carried that foundation forward.

She earned her bachelor's degree, then later went back for her master's while working at a university. For twenty-five years, she worked as a counselor helping students figure out how to get to college. She was educated, gainfully employed, and independent. She believed in preventative care. She went to her appointments. She followed recommendations. She trusted her healthcare team.

By every measure we usually use to explain poor health outcomes, Mary should not have been at risk.

And yet, she almost lost a decade of her life.

The phone calls started slowly. I was in California. She was in Indiana. At first, they were simple check-ins. Then they became frequent. Urgent. Sometimes multiple times a day. The tone shifted. The questions changed. She began needing help with things that had always come easily to her.

At work, she started struggling in ways that were impossible to ignore. She could not manage her email. She missed steps when planning events, even when I walked her through them. Her supervisor began asking for written responses. Listening from another state, I could hear what others around her did not seem to see. Something was wrong.

Mary had always been the one who managed health in her household. She raised three children. She kept track of appointments. She handled details. But now she is losing weight. She stopped cooking. She relied on nutritional supplements like Ensure to get through the day. At the time, that felt like a small adjustment. It was not.

The warning signs kept piling up.

She had multiple car incidents or fender-binders. Once, she could not reverse her car out of a parking space and asked a teenager to move it for her. Another time, she drove in the snow with a child in the backseat and was stopped by police who called EMS. At the hospital, they called me and told me her blood sugar was twenty. Normal is eighty to one hundred ten. They told me she weighed one hundred four pounds. She had previously been one hundred thirty-four.

Her gait was different, she started to drag her leg. Mary was going to physical therapy three times a week. She was going to the gym every morning before work. She kept trying to fix what she thought was a strength problem.

No one stepped back to ask the bigger question.

From across the country, I did.

I pushed for her to get time off. I pushed for her to get a disability leave, even when it was initially denied. I flew to Indiana because I needed to see it for myself. What I walked into was devastating. Her apartment was nearly unlivable. Ninety degrees inside. No food in the refrigerator. Floors that looked untouched for months.

That day, I bought two suitcases and told my aunt she was coming to live with me.

Back in California, everything changed. I brought her to my doctor. Specialists followed. She needed a hip replacement. She was diagnosed with Alzheimer's Disease. She was nearly blind in one eye. Surgeries were scheduled. Physical therapy followed.

She started walking again. Seeing again. Living again.

She is now healthier than she has been in years.

Mary did not ignore her health.

She did not avoid care.

She did not lack education.

She did not fail to try.

And still, she almost lost ten years of her life.

If this can happen to someone like Mary, what chance does someone have who does not have an advocate?

Someone who does not know what questions to ask?

Someone who assumes that showing up is enough?

Mary survived because I intervened.

Most people do not have a Carla.

This book is for them.

Across America, Black communities are losing ten years of life. Ten years. That is not a statistic. That is missed graduations, empty Sunday dinners, birthdays never celebrated, and weddings with brides walking without their fathers. It is a decade of dreams deferred, wisdom lost, and grief that compounds quietly.

Understanding the Lost Decade

When we talk about Black communities losing ten years of life, we are not speaking in metaphors or exaggerations. This loss is measured, documented, and felt in homes across the country. Ten years is not meant to shock. It is meant to show what families are missing.

A decade holds thousands of moments that shape a family. Advice given before adulthood. Laughter shared at Sunday dinners. Wisdom passed down in quiet conversations. When those years disappear, families lose more than time. They lose guidance, stability, and emotional inheritance.

The tragedy is that much of this loss is preventable.

It does not come from one dramatic event. It builds slowly through delayed diagnoses, unclear instructions, untreated conditions, and a healthcare system that often assumes understanding instead of ensuring it. The decade slips away in missed follow-ups, misunderstood symptoms, unmanaged diabetes, untreated hypertension, and misinformation that spreads faster than the truth.

This is the heart of the lost decade. The gap between what could have been lived and what was taken.

And at the center of that gap is healthcare literacy.

Healthcare literacy is the ability to understand, use, and act on health information. That's it. But when that ability is missing or inadequate, the consequences are deadly.

You can have access to care and still misunderstand a prescription label.

You can see a doctor and still leave confused.

You can receive a diagnosis and still make a life-altering decision because no one made sure you truly understood.

In over thirty years of nursing, from the steel town of Gary, Indiana, to executive boardrooms, I have watched this play out again and again. Patients blamed for noncompliance when no one took the time to explain. Families labeled as difficult when all they wanted was clarity. Lives shortened not by lack of care, but by lack of understanding.

This book is my call to action.

A map for anyone who has ever left a doctor's office overwhelmed.

A guide for families who want to protect the people they love.

A challenge to a system that too often equates information given with understanding received.

The Lost Decade does not just name the problem. It offers a way forward.

We will explore how history, culture, and communication collide to steal time year by year. We will talk honestly about the cost of low health literacy and then move into solutions: self-advocacy, community education, digital tools, and policy changes that can help reclaim what has been lost.

Because we cannot afford to keep losing time.

Not another year.

Not another life.
The decade is not gone yet.
We can still take it back.

WHO THIS BOOK IS FOR

This book is written first and foremost for patients.

It is for people sitting in exam rooms, listening carefully, nodding along, and later realizing they are not entirely sure what was just said. It is for people who want to do the right thing for their health but feel overwhelmed by medical language, rushed appointments, and decisions that seem bigger than the time they are given to make them.

If you have ever left a doctor's office with more questions than answers, this book is for you.

For Patients

Many patients enter healthcare spaces with courage and good intentions, yet leave with confusion. Not because they lack intelligence, effort, or concern for their health, but because the system often communicates in shorthand, assumptions, and time constraints.

A rushed explanation.

A crowded waiting room.

A provider moving quickly to the next appointment.

These moments stack up, leaving patients unsure about what is happening inside their own bodies and hesitant to speak up.

This book is designed to close that gap.

You will learn how to understand what is being said, how to ask clearer questions, and how to recognize when something does not feel right. You will gain language for conversations you may have avoided and insight into parts of the healthcare system that are rarely explained. The goal is not to make you a medical expert. The goal is to help you become an informed participant in your own care.

Because understanding is not a luxury. It is protection.

For Those Who Support Patients

While this book is written to patients, it will also be valuable for those who support them. Family members, friends, and loved ones often sit quietly in appointments, help manage follow-up care, or notice changes long before a provider does.

If you are reading this because you want to better support someone you love, this book will help you recognize warning signs, understand what questions matter most, and know when and how to speak up. Advocacy does not require medical training. It requires awareness, confidence, and clarity.

For Providers and Allies

This book is not written to critique providers, but many will recognize its value.

Healthcare works best when patients understand what is happening and feel confident enough to participate in their care. When patients have clarity, communication improves, follow-through increases, and trust has space to grow.

Providers who care deeply about outcomes will see how patient understanding changes the dynamic of care. Informed patients ask better questions, recognize early warning signs, and engage more meaningfully in decisions that affect their health.

This book supports that process by helping patients arrive prepared, informed, and empowered to take an active role in their care.

A Shared Commitment

Patients deserve information they can use.

Support systems deserve clarity about how to help.

Healthcare professionals deserve engaged, informed partners in care.

Reclaiming the lost decade is not about blame. It is about understanding, communication, and action. Everyone has a role to play, but it begins with ensuring that patients are never left in the dark about their own health.

WHAT'S AHEAD

The upcoming chapters will guide you through the subtle factors that have influenced health outcomes in Black communities for generations. You will see how history, policy, culture, and communication collide in ways that steal time, not all at once, but year by year, warning by ignored warning, and symptom by misunderstood symptom.

Because, sometimes data alone does not tell the full story, you will read stories from people I've personally spoken to who have been impacted by healthcare literacy or the lack of healthcare literacy they have. I'll share our talks and the strategies and tips we discussed to bridge the gap in healthcare literacy. These tips and strategies will be called **Dr. Carla's Caring Corner**. The purpose of this section is to address the statement I've unfortunately heard all too often, "I wish I would've known that" or "I had no idea." After reading this book, you and your loved ones will know these things, especially if you take the responsibility of each one, teach one.

Here's an inside track of what we will be covering in detail and the order in which we will be doing so. We begin by uncovering what health literacy really means and why it matters more than most people realize. You will learn how simple misunderstandings can become life-altering setbacks and why clarity is often the difference between early treatment and tragedy.

From there, we travel back through the medical scars left by betrayal and neglect. The past may be painful, but understanding it is the only way to rebuild trust. We will examine how those wounds continue to affect the choices families make today and why the medical system still struggles to connect with the communities that need it most.

We then move into the structural barriers that stand between Black patients and the care they deserve. Insurance, access, wait times, rushed visits, digital divides, the details matter, and each one carries a cost. You will see how these obstacles work together to delay diagnoses, complicate treatment, and shorten lives long before a doctor ever writes a prescription.

Later chapters shift from problems to solutions. You will learn practical strategies for advocating for yourself or someone you love, including the questions to ask, the mistakes to avoid, and the moments where speaking up can change the entire outcome. We will look at how communities can build their own literacy around health, technology, and prevention, even when resources are limited.

Finally, we explore what needs to change at the policy level so families are not forced to fight for clarity in a system built to be complex. You will witness the improvements, investments, and structural changes that can help restore the lost decade, not just theoretically but also practically.

By the end of this book, you'll know what's happening, why it's been going on for so long, what can be done about it now, and how patients, practitioners, and policymakers can reclaim lost years.

The goal is simple: more clarity, more confidence, and, more importantly, a decade reclaimed.

CHAPTER 1

Understanding Healthcare Literacy

Willie was a divorced, seventy-eight year old Black man who kept his health challenges to himself. Living alone and naturally quiet, his family never really knew what he was dealing with until the day he was diagnosed with colon cancer and needed surgery, a partial colectomy, to remove part of his colon.

The hospital's discharge planning made it clear: Willie couldn't care for himself in his weakened post-operative state. He would need a caregiver, even temporarily. So he went to recuperate at his son and daughter-in-law's home, and for a while, things looked promising. Willie showed signs of recovery. His activity level increased, and his appetite returned. He seemed to be on his way back to health.

Then one day, his daughter-in-law came home from work to find her husband sitting alone on the sofa. "Where is dad?"

she asked. Her husband explained that his brother had come to visit, and Willie had gone to the bathroom. When he took too long to return, they went to check on him and found him dead.

Up until Willie's death, his son had been putting off his own colonoscopy despite his wife's urging. It wasn't until he lost his father to colon cancer that the reality hit home, this was now a documented risk factor in his family history that he could no longer ignore. When he finally got his first colonoscopy, they removed several polyps that could have become cancerous.

Willie's story isn't unique, and it's not just about older men. During a community tour of a prison, visitors stopped at a large auditorium where half a dozen incarcerated men, all minorities, stood before the audience answering random questions. Nothing was off limits. Suddenly, a nurse in the back stood up and asked, "Why do so many of you refuse your colon screenings while you're here in prison?"

The answer came later when the tour resumed. A prisoner pulled the nurse aside and said, "We don't want to be violated." Prison rape is real, and the threat of forcible rectal penetration is something many of these men live in fear of. When the nurse pressed for clarification, it became clear that this man believed the colonoscopy procedure was painful, violating, humiliating, and performed while awake.

The reality? Colonoscopies are performed under sedation. When you wake up, you have absolutely no memory of the procedure, no rectal pain, not even a hint that a scope entered your rectum. The fears are unfounded and based on ignorance, ignorance that is robbing Black men of a decade of life to undiagnosed colon cancer.

DEFINING HEALTHCARE LITERACY

Let's be honest, when you walk into a doctor's office, do you ever feel like everyone's speaking a different language? Like they're using words that sound like English but might as well be ancient Greek? You're not alone, and you're not "slow" for feeling this way. Healthcare literacy is about having the power to understand and use health information to make decisions about your care. But really, it's about not feeling lost in your own health journey.

You might think healthcare literacy is just about reading those tiny labels on your prescription bottles trying to figure out if you're supposed to take two pills in the morning or one pill twice a day. Sure, that's part of it. But if that's all it was, we wouldn't have millions of people leaving doctor's appointments confused, scared, and no closer to getting better. Healthcare literacy is like having a translator for a system that seems determined to keep you in the dark.

Think about the last time a doctor threw medical terms at you. Maybe they said you have "moderate persistent asthma with acute exacerbation." You might have nodded along, but inside you're thinking: "Is this serious? Am I dying? Can I still play basketball with my kids?" Healthcare literacy means knowing that your doctor just told you your breathing problems are getting worse and could land you in the emergency room if you don't get them under control. More importantly, it means feeling confident enough to stop them and say, "Break that down for me doc. What exactly does that mean for my daily life?"

Every time you deal with health insurance, you need healthcare literacy. You know those forms that ask about deductibles, co-insurance, and out-of-pocket maximums? They're not trying to confuse you on purpose (though it might feel that way). When you understand that your deductible is what you pay before insurance kicks in, suddenly you realize why that MRI costs you $1,200 in January but only $200 in November. When you see "prior authorization required," you know it means your doctor needs to argue with your insurance company, that it's not your fault, and you didn't mess up.

The real-world consequences of limited healthcare literacy can be devastating. When you don't understand medical procedures, when misinformation fills the gaps in your knowledge, when fear prevents you from getting life-saving care, you become vulnerable to outcomes like Willie's.

Think about those incarcerated men refusing colonoscopies because they believed the procedure would be violating and painful. Their fear wasn't based on medical reality, it was based on misinformation and assumptions. They didn't understand that colonoscopies are performed under sedation, that patients have no memory of the procedure, that there's no pain or awareness during the screening. This gap in healthcare literacy literally prevented them from accessing care that could save their lives.

Willie himself may have avoided routine screening for years because he didn't understand the importance of early detection. Maybe he thought colonoscopies were only for people who were already sick. Maybe he didn't know that colon cancer screening guidelines recommend starting at age 45 for Black men because we face higher rates and earlier onset. His family didn't know about his health challenges because he kept them private, possibly out of shame or fear that came from not understanding his conditions or treatment options.

Here's what changes when you have healthcare literacy: You walk into that doctor's office like it's your space too. When they say your blood pressure is 140 over 90, you don't just nod, you ask, "What can I do to fix this before we talk about pills?" When they prescribe something new, you ask about side effects, how long you'll need to take it, and what happens if you can't afford it. You're not being difficult; you're being smart about your health.

At the pharmacy counter, you know you can ask questions. "Is there a generic version?" "What happens if I miss a dose?" "Will this mess with my other medications?" The pharmacist isn't judging you, answering your questions is literally their job. When your insurance denies something, you know you can fight back. You can appeal. You can ask your doctor to try again. You're not helpless.

Without healthcare literacy, every medical situation feels like walking through a minefield blindfolded. You leave appointments confused but too embarrassed to call back for clarification. You get prescriptions filled but take them wrong or stop taking them when you feel better, not knowing you're supposed to finish the whole course. Bills show up that make no sense, so you either pay too much or throw them in a drawer until a collection agency starts calling. You miss follow-up appointments because nobody explained why they mattered.

For you, for your family, for your community, healthcare literacy isn't just about understanding medical terms. It's about survival in a system that wasn't designed with you in mind. It's about knowing enough to spot the difference between good medical advice and the misleading health information flooding your Facebook feed and family group chats. It's about having the confidence to advocate for yourself when you know something's not right, even when they're trying to dismiss your concerns.

You deserve to understand what's happening with your body. You deserve answers that make sense, not medical riddles, and you absolutely deserve to be an equal partner in your healthcare, not a confused bystander watching your own life happen to you.

THE THREE LEVELS OF HEALTH LITERACY

Understanding healthcare isn't like learning to drive, where you either have a license or you don't. Health literacy exists on three different levels, and where you fall on this spectrum can literally determine how many healthy years you have left. For Black Americans, these gaps in health literacy aren't just personal shortcomings, they're part of a larger pattern that's stealing a decade of life from our communities. Let's break down what each level looks like and why it matters for your survival in the healthcare system.

Level 1: Basic Health Literacy

Basic health literacy is your foundation, can you read and understand basic health information? This sounds simple until you're sitting in a doctor's office trying to make sense of a discharge summary that says you have "acute myocardial infarction with subsequent cardiac rehabilitation recommended." Even if you can read every word, do you understand they're telling you that you had a heart attack and need to start a specific exercise program?

You might think basic literacy issues are rare, but the truth is shocking. Nearly 90 million Americans, that's more than 1 in 3 adults struggle with basic health literacy. According to the National Assessment of Adult Literacy, only 12% of adults have proficient health literacy skills, with significantly lower rates in Black and Hispanic communities. In our communities, this number is even higher due to decades of educational inequity and healthcare systems that assume everyone speaks "medical English."

Remember Willie from our opening story? His quiet nature and tendency to keep health issues private might have stemmed partly from limited health literacy. When doctors used terms like "partial colectomy" or explained his post-operative care requirements, did he fully understand what they meant? Did he know what warning signs to watch for during recovery? His family didn't know about his health challenges, which suggests he may not have had the literacy skills to explain his condition clearly or advocate for additional support.

This level impacts every single interaction with the healthcare system. Insurance cards filled with abbreviations like "PCP," "HMO," and "Rx" become meaningless puzzles. Medication bottles with warnings about "drowsiness" or "photosensitivity" leave people guessing whether they should avoid driving or going outside. Even something as basic as understanding that "PRN" means "as needed" can be the difference between proper pain management and accidental overdose.

When you can't read or understand basic health information, you're forced to rely entirely on what healthcare providers tell you and hope they're looking out for your best interests. You can't verify information, can't research your conditions, and can't advocate for alternatives. This makes you vulnerable to both poor care and missed opportunities for life-saving interventions.

Level 2: Functional Health Literacy

Functional health literacy takes things up a notch. You can read the words, but can you apply that information to your specific situation? Can you take what the doctor told you and actually use it to improve your health? This is where the rubber meets the road, and it's where many people hit a wall.

Take diabetes management. Your doctor says to "check your blood sugar before meals and adjust your insulin accordingly." You understand each word, but applying this to real life is complicated. What counts as a meal? What if you're working double shifts and eating at irregular times? How do you adjust insulin when the directions say "sliding scale" but nobody explains what that scale actually looks like for your body weight and activity level?

Functional health literacy also affects how you navigate the healthcare system itself. You might understand that you need a referral to see a specialist, but do you know that some insurance plans require you to get that referral from your primary care doctor first, while others let you go directly? Do you understand that "in-network" versus "out-of-network" can mean the difference between a $30 copay and a $500 bill?

Consider the incarcerated men who refused colonoscopies. They had enough basic literacy to understand that the procedure involved rectal examination, but they lacked the functional literacy to understand what the procedure actually entailed. They couldn't process the information that colonoscopies are performed under sedation or that patients have no awareness during the procedure. Their functional health literacy gap turned a life-saving screening into something they feared and avoided.

This level of literacy also determines whether you can follow through with treatment plans. You might understand that physical therapy will help your back pain, but if you don't understand that insurance typically covers only a limited number of sessions, you might stop going when your copays start adding up, thinking you can't afford to continue. Meanwhile, your condition gets worse, leading to more expensive interventions later.

Level 3: Critical Health Literacy

Critical health literacy is the highest level. This is where you become the CEO of your own health. You don't just read and apply health information; you evaluate it, question it, and make informed decisions. You can spot the difference between reliable medical advice and the health misinformation that floods social media. In our communities, where mistrust of the medical system runs deep for good historical reasons, this level of literacy becomes crucial for survival.

Critical health literacy means you can look at treatment options and make informed choices. When your doctor recommends surgery for your prostate cancer, you know to ask about active surveillance, radiation therapy, and surgical options. You understand that "watchful waiting" might sound scary, but for some cancers, it's actually the safest approach. You know to ask about success rates, side effects, and how the decision might affect your quality of life.

But here's where it gets complicated for Black Americans: Critical health literacy also means being able to advocate for yourself in a system that often doesn't advocate for you. When your doctor dismisses your chest pain as anxiety, you know that Black women are significantly more likely to have heart attacks misdiagnosed. You push for an EKG, stress test, or cardiology referral because you understand that your symptoms deserve the same thorough evaluation anyone else would receive.

Willie's son demonstrated critical health literacy when he finally understood that his father's colon cancer created a family history risk factor that he couldn't ignore. He had the critical thinking skills to connect his father's death to his own health risks and to overcome whatever hesitation he had about getting screened. When they found and removed polyps during his first colonoscopy, his critical health literacy likely saved his life.

Critical health literacy also means being able to evaluate health information critically. When your cousin shares an article claiming that baking soda cures cancer, you know to check if the source is a peer-reviewed medical journal or a wellness blog trying to sell supplements. When a video goes viral claiming vaccines cause diabetes, you understand how to look up the actual research and see that diabetes rates in unvaccinated populations are actually higher.

This level of literacy becomes life-or-death when dealing with misinformation that specifically targets our communities. You can recognize when social media posts prey on historical medical trauma to discourage preventive care. You understand that while systemic racism in healthcare is real, refusing all medical treatment isn't the answer but finding providers you trust and being an informed advocate for yourself is.

The tragic reality is that many people in our communities never reach this level of critical health literacy, not because they're not smart enough, but because the healthcare system actively works against patient empowerment. Doctors who are rushed or who carry unconscious biases don't take the time to ensure understanding. Insurance systems are deliberately complicated to discourage utilization. Medical information is often presented in ways that discourage questioning rather than encourage partnership.

But here's what happens when you develop critical health literacy: You stop being a passive recipient of healthcare and become an active participant. You ask questions that matter. You seek second opinions when something doesn't feel right. You research your conditions and come to appointments prepared. You understand that your health outcomes are too important to leave entirely in someone else's hands.

The difference between these three levels isn't just academic, it's the difference between surviving and thriving, between catching diseases early and dying from preventable complications. In our communities, where we're already fighting against shorter life expectancies and higher disease rates, healthcare literacy isn't just helpful, it's essential for reclaiming those lost years.

HOW HEALTH LITERACY CORRELATES WITH LIFE EXPECTANCY

Here's a number that should make you angry: Black Americans live, on average, 10 years less than white Americans. Ten years. That's a decade of watching grandchildren grow up, of retirement you'll never see, of dreams you'll never fulfill. While racism, poverty, and systemic healthcare failures all play roles in this gap, there's one factor that doesn't get enough attention, healthcare literacy. The inability to understand and navigate the healthcare system is literally stealing years from your life, and it's time you understood exactly how this happens.

Those 10 years aren't just numbers on a government report. They represent real people in your family, your neighborhood, your church. They're Willie, who died during recovery from colon cancer surgery. They're the incarcerated men who refuse life-saving colonoscopies because they don't understand what the procedure actually involves. They're your uncle who died at 58 from a heart attack that could have been prevented if he'd understood that chest pain during exercise meant "go to the ER now," not "tough it out until Monday."

The Chronic Disease Pipeline

Limited health literacy creates a direct pipeline to chronic disease, and here's how it works: You don't understand the early warning signs, so you miss the window for prevention. You don't understand your diagnosis, so you can't manage it properly. You don't understand your treatment, so the condition gets worse until it becomes life-threatening.

Take hypertension, the "silent killer", that affects nearly half of all Black adults. When your doctor says your blood pressure is 140/90 and you need to "watch your sodium intake," limited health literacy means you might stop adding salt to your food but continue eating processed meals loaded with hidden sodium. You don't understand that the chicken sandwich from your favorite restaurant has more sodium than you should eat in an entire day. You don't know that "low sodium" on a label still might be too high for someone with high blood pressure.

Diabetes tells an even starker story. In our communities, Type 2 Diabetes isn't just common, it's an epidemic. But here's what limited health literacy does: It makes Diabetes management feel impossible instead of manageable. When your doctor says to "count carbs," but you don't understand that rice, bread, and fruit all count as carbohydrates, you're set up for failure from day one. When they prescribe metformin and say it might cause stomach upset, but don't explain that taking it with food helps and the side effects usually improve, you might stop taking it and never tell your doctor.

The Early Detection Crisis

Healthcare literacy fundamentally determines whether diseases are caught early when they're treatable, or late when they're deadly. This isn't just about scheduling regular checkups, it's about understanding what those tests mean and why they matter before you feel sick.

Consider colon cancer screening, the exact type of preventive care that could have saved Willie's life. The guidelines changed to recommend colonoscopies starting at age 45 for Black Americans instead of 50, because we face higher rates and earlier onset. But limited health literacy means many people don't understand that this change applies to them, don't understand why they need screening when they feel fine, or don't understand what the procedure actually involves.

The incarcerated men in our opening story represent thousands of Black men who avoid this life-saving screening because of misinformation and fear. They believed the procedure would be violating and painful, not understanding that patients are sedated and have no memory or sensation during colonoscopy. This health literacy gap widens when patients are not aware of the facts about a common medical procedure which keeps men from getting screened until symptoms appear, when treatment is more difficult and survival rates are lower.

Willie's son finally got screened after his father's death, and they found and removed polyps that could have become cancerous. If Willie had understood the importance of regular screening, if he'd had the health literacy to ask about family history and risk factors, if he'd known that early detection dramatically improves survival rates, he might still be alive today.

The same pattern plays out with mammograms, where Black women are more likely to die from breast cancer despite having slightly lower incidence rates. Part of this comes from limited health literacy around breast health. Many women don't understand that dense breast tissue (more common in Black women) can hide tumors on mammograms, meaning they might need additional screening like ultrasounds or MRIs. They don't know to ask about their breast density or what it means for their screening schedule.

The Medication Management Disaster

Poor health literacy turns prescription medications from life-savers into potential hazards. It's not just about reading the label, it's about understanding how medications work, why you need to take them even when you feel better, and what to do when something doesn't seem right.

Blood pressure medications offer a perfect example. Limited health literacy leads people to think these medications are like antibiotics. You take them until you feel better, then you stop. But blood pressure medicine works only as long as you take it. When you feel better and stop taking it, your blood pressure goes right back up, often higher than before.

Medication interactions represent another health literacy crisis. People don't understand that their supplements, over-the-counter medications, and prescriptions can interact in dangerous ways. They don't know that grapefruit can make some heart medications toxic, some cough medicine can raise your blood pressure, or that ibuprofen can interfere with blood pressure medications.

The Fear and Misinformation Factor

Willie's story illustrates how health literacy gaps create space for fear and misinformation to flourish. The incarcerated men who refused colonoscopies weren't making informed decisions, they were making fear-based decisions rooted in misinformation. They didn't understand the reality of the procedure, so their minds filled in the gaps with worst-case scenarios.

This pattern repeats across healthcare. When people don't understand medical procedures, treatments, or diagnoses, fear and misinformation rush in to fill the void. Social media amplifies these fears, sharing horror stories and conspiracy theories that prey on legitimate concerns about racism in healthcare. Without strong health literacy skills, it becomes impossible to separate valid concerns from dangerous misinformation.

The result is that people avoid life-saving care, stop taking necessary medications, or turn to unproven alternative treatments. Each avoided screening, each missed diagnosis, each untreated condition steals time from lives that are already statistically shorter than they should be.

The Healthcare System Complexity Trap

The healthcare system's complexity punishes people with limited health literacy. When you need to see a specialist, limited health literacy means you might not understand that you need a referral from your primary care doctor first. When your insurance requires "prior authorization" for a medication, you might think you've done something wrong rather than understanding this is a cost-control mechanism. When you receive medical bills, you might pay the full amount rather than understanding "allowable amounts" or how to navigate insurance processing and appeals.

Each of these literacy gaps creates barriers to care, delays in treatment, and additional financial stress that further discourages healthcare utilization. The system seems designed to reward those who can navigate its complexity while punishing those who cannot.

Can Health Literacy Alone Close the Gap?

Here's the truth: Improving health literacy alone won't eliminate the 10-year life expectancy gap between Black and white Americans. Racism in healthcare, poverty, environmental factors, and systemic inequities all play crucial roles. Health literacy is one factor you can control, and it amplifies the effect of every other intervention.

When you have strong health literacy, you're better equipped to navigate a racist healthcare system. You know what questions to ask when a doctor dismisses your symptoms. You understand when you need to seek a second opinion and that it is your right. You can identify quality healthcare providers and avoid ones who don't serve your community well.

Health literacy also helps you make the most of whatever healthcare access you have. Even if you can only afford to see a doctor once a year, strong health literacy helps you prepare for that appointment, ask the right questions, and understand the guidance you receive. It helps you recognize which symptoms require immediate attention versus which ones can wait for your next appointment.

But let's be clear: The healthcare system's complexity isn't an accident. Insurance companies benefit when people don't understand their coverage and pay more than they should. Some healthcare providers benefit when patients don't ask questions or seek second opinions. Pharmaceutical companies benefit when people don't understand generic alternatives, prescription apps or manufacturer assistance programs.

This means that while improving your health literacy can add years to your life, we also need systemic changes: healthcare providers trained in clear communication, insurance systems designed for transparency rather than confusion, and medical information presented in ways that empower rather than intimidate.

Your Health Literacy as Life Insurance

Think of health literacy as life insurance that you pay for with time and effort instead of money. Every hour you spend learning about your conditions, understanding your medications, and navigating the healthcare system is an investment in additional years of life.

Willie's son learned this lesson too late to save his father, but not too late to save himself. When he finally understood the connection between his father's colon cancer and his own risk, he got screened and caught polyps before they became cancerous. His health literacy, gained through tragic experience, likely added years to his life.

The 10-year gap in life expectancy isn't destiny, it's a problem with solutions. While you can't single-handedly fix systemic racism or healthcare inequity, you can arm yourself with the knowledge and skills to navigate the system more effectively. You can learn to be an advocate for your own health, to spot misinformation before it derails your care, and to make informed decisions even in a system that wasn't designed with your success in mind.

Those 10 years? They're not gone forever. With better health literacy, earlier detection, proper medication management, and effective advocacy, you can reclaim them. The question isn't whether the healthcare system will change overnight, it won't. The question is whether you'll develop the tools to thrive within it while fighting to make it better.

Your life depends on it. Literally.

CLOSING THOUGHTS

If you've made it this far, you now understand something that many healthcare professionals don't fully grasp: Healthcare literacy isn't just about reading comprehension or education level. It's about power, advocacy, and survival in a system that often seems designed to keep you confused and dependent. But here's what most people miss about healthcare literacy, it's not a personal failing when you don't understand medical jargon or can't navigate insurance bureaucracy. The system is broken, not you.

The Most Overlooked Truth

The most overlooked aspect of healthcare literacy isn't what you don't know, it's how the healthcare system actively works against your understanding. Think about it: If hospitals and insurance companies really wanted you to understand your care, would they send you home with discharge papers written at a high-school reading level? Would they design insurance plans with dozens of confusing terms and hidden costs? Would they schedule 15-minute appointments for physicals, and complex chronic diseases that require lifestyle changes?

The uncomfortable truth is that patient confusion is profitable. When you don't understand your insurance benefits, you might pay for services that should be covered. When you don't understand your treatment options, you're more likely to accept expensive procedures without questioning alternatives. When you don't understand prevention, you end up needing costly emergency interventions later. Poor health literacy costs the U.S. healthcare system an estimated $106-238 billion annually, money that comes out of higher premiums, increased taxes, and inflated medical costs that affect everyone.

This isn't a conspiracy, it's a business model and recognizing this truth is the first step toward protecting yourself and your family. You're not struggling with healthcare literacy because you're not smart enough. You're struggling because you're navigating a system that benefits from your confusion.

What Needs to Change First

If we could wave a magic wand and fix one aspect of the healthcare system to make it more accessible, it should be communication. Imagine if every healthcare interaction was designed around one simple question: "Does the patient truly understand what we just told them, and do they feel confident acting on this information?"

Picture walking out of a doctor's appointment with a one-page summary written in plain language that explains: what's wrong with you, what you need to do about it, when you need to do it, what to watch for, and when to call for help. No medical jargon, no confusing abbreviations, just clear information you can share with your family and refer back to when you're at home trying to remember what the doctor said.

Imagine if those incarcerated men had received clear, accurate information about colonoscopies and that the procedure is performed under sedation, that patients have no memory or sensation during the screening, and that it's the most effective way to prevent colon cancer deaths. How many Black lives could have been saved with just better communication about what the procedure actually involves?

Imagine insurance cards that actually make sense, where "deductible" and "out-of-pocket maximum" are explained in everyday terms, where you can easily see what services are covered and what they'll cost you. Imagine prescription labels that include not just dosing instructions, but why you're taking this medication, what it's supposed to do, and what to expect.

This isn't fantasy, other countries have implemented clearer healthcare communication standards. The Netherlands requires all patient information to be written at a 6th-grade reading level. Australia has "Ask Me 3" campaigns that encourage patients to ask three specific questions at every appointment: What is my main problem? What do I need to do? Why is it important for me to do this?

What's Already Working

Despite the system's flaws, there are bright spots, programs and strategies that are successfully improving health literacy in communities like ours. Community health workers, often called "promotoras" in Latino communities or "community health workers" in Black communities, are making real differences. These are people from your neighborhood who receive training to help others navigate the healthcare system, understand their conditions, and advocate for themselves.

Churches and community centers are hosting health literacy workshops that teach practical skills: how to read medication labels, how to prepare for doctor's appointments, and how to understand insurance benefits. The key is that these programs meet people where they are, both literally and culturally. They're taught by people who look like you, who understand your experiences, and who can translate medical information into language that makes sense in your daily life.

Some healthcare systems are also stepping up. Kaiser Permanente has implemented "health literacy universal precautions". They assume every patient might have limited health literacy and design all their communications accordingly. They use plain language, visual aids, and teach-back methods where they ask patients to repeat back what they've learned to ensure understanding.

Technology is also creating new opportunities. Apps like "Ask Me 3: Good Questions for Your Good Health" remind you to ask key questions during appointments. Medication reminder apps don't just tell you when to take pills, they explain why you're taking them and what to expect. Telehealth platforms are creating space for longer, more detailed conversations about care.

The Road Forward

Healthcare providers need to fundamentally change how they think about patient education. Instead of viewing it as an add-on service they provide when time allows, it needs to become central to every interaction. Medical schools need to teach future doctors how to communicate clearly, how to recognize when patients don't understand, and how to explain complex concepts in accessible ways. This is particularly true for the carceral population.

Educators at all levels need to integrate health literacy into the curriculum. Your child should graduate high school knowing how insurance works, what preventive care means, and how to advocate for themselves in medical settings. This isn't just health class, this is life skills education that could add years to their lives.

Policymakers need to stop treating health literacy as a nice-to-have and start treating it as a matter of life and death. Insurance regulations should require clear, standardized language. Hospital accreditation should depend partly on patient comprehension rates, not just clinical outcomes. Public health funding should prioritize health literacy programs in communities with the worst health outcomes.

But here's what you can't wait for: You can't wait for the system to change to start improving your own health literacy. You can't wait for your doctor to get better at explaining things to start asking better questions. You can't wait for your insurance company to simplify their plans to start understanding your current coverage.

Your Power in This Moment

Think back to Willie's story. What could have saved him? Better communication about post-operative warning signs. Family health literacy that encouraged him to share his health challenges rather than keeping them private. Earlier screening that caught his cancer before surgery was needed. Understanding of family risk factors that motivated his son to get screened sooner.

Willie's son learned too late to save his father, but not too late to save himself. When he finally understood the connection between his father's death and his own risk factors, he took action. His health literacy, tragic though its source was, likely added years to his life when they found and removed those polyps.

The incarcerated men who refused colonoscopies based on misinformation represent a different tragedy because they are preventable deaths that could be avoided with better health education. Their fears weren't unreasonable given their life experiences, but they were uninformed. With accurate information about what colonoscopy actually involves, many of those men could make informed decisions that save their lives.

The remainder of this book will give you specific tools, strategies, and resources to build your health literacy skills. You'll learn how to identify reliable health information in an age of misinformation. You'll discover how to prepare for medical appointments to get the most out of them. You'll understand how to navigate insurance, medication management, and advocacy in ways that can literally save your life.

Before we get to those practical skills, remember this: Every time you ask a question, every time you seek clarification, every time you refuse to leave a medical appointment confused, you're not just improving your own health outcomes, you're helping to change the system. Healthcare providers learn to communicate better when patients demand better communication. Insurance companies simplify their processes when customers refuse to accept confusion.

You have more power than you realize. The same critical thinking skills that help you spot a scam phone call can help you identify health misinformation. The same determination that helps you advocate for your children can help you advocate for your own healthcare. The same community connections that sustain you through other challenges can become resources for better health literacy.

Those 10 years the healthcare system is trying to steal from you? They're not gone yet. With better health literacy, you can fight for them. With stronger advocacy skills, you can reclaim them. With a clearer understanding of how the system works, you can navigate it successfully despite its flaws.

The journey toward better health literacy isn't just about individual improvement, it's about community empowerment. When you understand your health better, you can help your family understand theirs. When you learn to navigate the system effectively, you can guide others through it. When you develop skills to spot misinformation, you can protect your community from dangerous health myths.

This is how change happens: one person, one family, one community at a time, refusing to accept confusion as normal and demanding the clear, respectful healthcare communication you deserve. Your health literacy isn't just about you, it's about all of us reclaiming those lost years together.

TIPS FROM DR. CARLA'S CARING CORNER

- Polyps are known to be a precursor to cancer. Count your blessings if they are found and removed.
- Higher rates of colon cancer exist among Blacks. Our ignorance, fear of screening, and oftentimes complacency can and often does result in many lost decades.
- Ask your primary doctor to refer you to a gastroenterologist who specializes in disease of the alimentary canal or mouth to rectum. It is this discipline that performs colonoscopies.
- Always inform your doctor of bowel changes, prolonged constipation or diarrhea, rectal bleeding, poop that is black or tarry looking, drainage from your navel as these could be signs of disease.

CHAPTER 2

The Historical Betrayal – Mistrust in the Medical System

You might be wondering why your grandmother clutches her purse and not her pearls tighter when she walks into a doctor's office. Why does your uncle keep putting off that surgery his doctor says he needs. Why do you feel a knot in your stomach every time you have to go to the hospital?

It's not paranoia. It's not ignorance. It's survival instinct built on generations of betrayal.

When Black folks say they don't trust the healthcare system, we're not being difficult. We're remembering. If you've ever felt like you can't fully trust the doctor across from you, this chapter will help you understand why. It will also show you that while your mistrust is completely justified, it doesn't have to control your healthcare decisions or cost you years of your life.

WHEN MEDICINE BECAME THE ENEMY

The betrayal didn't start recently. It's been building for generations, each violation adding another layer to the wall between our communities and the healthcare system.

The Tuskegee Nightmare

In 1932, the U.S. Department of Public Health, working with the Tuskegee Institute in Alabama, began what they called a study of "bad blood" in Black men. Six hundred men participated, 400 who had syphilis and 200 who didn't. These men thought they were getting free healthcare, free meals, and burial insurance.

The researchers never told the men they had syphilis. Even after penicillin became the standard cure for syphilis in the 1940s (a cure that was widely available by 1948) the men in the study were deliberately denied treatment. For forty years, doctors watched these men suffer, go blind, lose their minds, and die, all so they could observe how untreated syphilis destroys the human body.

One hundred men died. Their wives got infected. Their children were born with the disease. All while doctors with the power to save them took notes instead.

The Women They Tortured

James Marion Sims, often called "the father of modern gynecology," built his reputation by operating on enslaved Black women without the benefit of anesthesia. Sims believed that Black women couldn't feel pain the same way white women could. This lie allowed him to cut into woman after woman, practicing procedures that would later make him famous and wealthy.

The most heartbreaking part? Some of those beliefs about Black women and pain still exist today. I've seen it throughout my career. Black women's pain dismissed or minimized in ways that would never happen to white patients. Studies show that some healthcare providers still believe Black patients have higher pain tolerance. None of it is true, but the bias is real.

The Woman Whose Cells Changed Medicine

In 1951, Henrietta Lacks went to Johns Hopkins Hospital for a lump that had been overlooked during her five previous childbirths. While treating her cervical cancer, doctors took samples of her cells without asking for permission, without telling her, and without explaining what they would be used for.

Those cells, later called HeLa cells, became the foundation for developing the polio vaccine, cancer treatments, and countless other medical breakthroughs that saved millions of lives and generated billions of dollars.

Henrietta died at age 31. Her family didn't learn about the cells until more than 20 years later. They weren't compensated. They weren't credited. For decades, they couldn't even afford the healthcare that was being developed using their mother's body.

The Bodies They Stole

In the 1960s, southern medical schools commonly dug up Black bodies from graves to use for teaching and research. Black families would bury their loved ones, only to have medical students later exhume and mutilate those bodies for practice.

You couldn't even trust that your loved ones would rest in peace. This isn't ancient history. Your grandparents and great-grandparents knew people who lived through this.

THE TRAUMA THAT LIVES IN OUR BODIES

When I talk to older patients, I see how this history shapes every interaction. This is generational trauma where the way pain and mistrust get passed down like family recipes. Your grandmother might not have told you the specific stories, but she taught you to be careful around doctors.

Maybe she told you things like:

- "Don't trust them white doctors" or "blue-eyed devils"
- "They experiment on people like us"
- "They don't care about Black folks"

These weren't just opinions. These were survival strategies based on real experiences.

Willie's story from Chapter 1 reflects this. His quiet nature and tendency to keep his health problems private might have been rooted in this kind of mistrust. Maybe he figured it was safer to handle things on his own rather than risk becoming another medical statistic.

HOW BETRAYAL SHOWS UP TODAY

The betrayal continues just in more subtle ways. Black patients are less likely to receive adequate pain medication. We're more likely to be labeled as "drug-seeking" when we report pain. Black women are three to four times more likely to die during childbirth than white women, even when you control for income and education.

We're underrepresented in medical research, which means treatments are developed and tested primarily on white bodies.

Our symptoms are more likely to be attributed to lifestyle factors rather than actual medical conditions.

Those incarcerated men from Willie's story who refused colonoscopies? Their refusal wasn't just based on misinformation, it was based on a deep, justified fear that the medical system would use their vulnerability against them.

THE COST OF MISTRUST

This broken trust is literally killing us. When you don't trust the system, you delay seeking care until conditions become life-threatening. Every day of delayed care, every avoided screening, every prescription that doesn't get filled all add up to shorter lives.

Here's what's tragic: while our mistrust is completely justified, the diseases don't care about our history. Cancer doesn't skip Black bodies because we've been experimented on. Heart disease doesn't give us a pass because our ancestors were betrayed.

BUILDING TRUST WITHOUT FORGETTING HISTORY

So where does this leave you? How do you protect yourself from a system that has a documented history of harming people who look like you, while still getting the healthcare you need?

The answer isn't to forget history. The answer is to use that history to become a smarter, more strategic healthcare consumer. Your awareness of these issues isn't paranoia, it's preparation.

Throughout my career, I've worked to rebuild trust, one patient at a time. I never tell patients their concerns about medical racism are invalid. Instead, I acknowledge their concerns and then show them how to navigate the system more safely.

Here's what I've learned works:

Find providers who acknowledge the history. If a doctor gets defensive when you mention concerns about medical racism, find another doctor. Good healthcare providers understand this history and work to overcome it.

Bring an advocate. Research shows that patients who bring someone with them receive better care. Having a witness changes how providers behave.

Ask questions and take notes. Don't let anyone rush you or make you feel stupid for seeking clarification.

Seek second opinions for major decisions. This protects you from potential bias or errors.

Know your family history and track your symptoms. The more prepared you are, the harder it is for providers to dismiss your concerns.

THE PATH FORWARD

The healthcare system owes our communities concrete changes that address the ongoing effects of historical betrayal. We need more Black healthcare providers, more community health centers, and more research that includes our experiences.

While we're fighting for these systemic changes, we can't wait for the system to fix itself before we take care of our health. Your mistrust of the medical system isn't wrong, it's rational. But that mistrust has to evolve from "stay away" to "engage strategically."

You can honor the lessons your family taught you about being careful while still getting the care you need. Your ancestors survived medical abuse so that you could be here today. Honor their sacrifice by taking care of yourself, but do it wisely.

The lost decade isn't just about healthcare literacy, it's also about the weight of history. Understanding that weight and learning how to carry it strategically can help you reclaim the healthy years that are rightfully yours.

You deserve healthcare that sees your humanity and prioritizes your wellbeing. The fact that the system has failed to provide this consistently doesn't mean you should go without care. It means you need to be smarter about how you get it.

Your mistrust was meant to protect you, use it as a tool for better healthcare, not as a barrier to getting any healthcare at all.

TIPS FROM DR. CARLA'S CARING CORNER

- Invite a doctoral prepared nurse to speak at your events so patients are armed with ethically sound information and education.
- Find healthcare staff that represent your culture and community. They are more likely to hear and validate your concerns.
- The International Review Board (IRB) exists to govern research and has stringent rules and guidelines around research on human subjects. The Tuskegee Syphilis Experiment won't happen again.
- Nothing can be done to you without your consent and it must be in writing.

CHAPTER 3

Systemic Barriers That Keep Black People in the Dark

Have you ever wondered why it feels like the healthcare system is designed to keep you confused? Like every form is written in a foreign language, every explanation comes too fast, and every resource you need is just out of reach?

You're not imagining it. When our communities don't have access to clear, accurate, and timely health information, the consequences are devastating. Not just confusion. Not just delay. Death.

This lack of access doesn't happen by accident. There are systems in place that are layered, longstanding, and often invisible that keep Black people in the dark. Systems that shape what we're taught, how we're treated, and how much we're able to trust what we hear.

So if you're wondering why we haven't "just figured it out by now," the answer is simple: we were never meant to. The barriers keeping you from understanding and navigating healthcare weren't created by coincidence. They were built into the system, and understanding them is the first step to breaking through them.

WHEN SCHOOLS FAIL TO TEACH WHAT MATTERS

If you don't learn it in school, where are you supposed to learn it? In too many Black communities, health education is either outdated, inconsistent, or altogether absent. I'm not talking about the one week of "reproductive health" that someone's gym teacher mumbled through in tenth grade. I'm talking about basic, lifelong knowledge: what blood pressure numbers mean, how to manage chronic illness, when to get screened for cancer, why symptoms matter.

That's not ignorance when people don't know these things. That's neglect. That's a system failing to teach people what they need to survive.

The health education gap starts early and compounds over time. While schools in affluent areas might have comprehensive health curricula, updated textbooks, advanced technology and school nurses on staff, schools in predominantly Black communities often struggle with basic resources. Health class becomes an afterthought, taught by whoever has a free period rather than by qualified health educators.

Even when health education exists, it's often disconnected from the realities of our communities. Students learn about diseases they've never heard of while getting no information about conditions that run in their families. They memorize the food pyramid while living in food deserts where fresh vegetables cost more than processed meals.

By the time you graduate high school, you might know the parts of a cell but not understand that high blood pressure runs in families and requires monitoring. You might know about photosynthesis but not that diabetes can cause blindness if left untreated. You learn biology but not practical health management.

This educational gap doesn't just affect individuals, it affects entire families. When parents don't understand health concepts, they can't teach their children. When teenagers don't learn about preventive care, they become adults who only seek medical attention in emergencies. The cycle perpetuates itself, generation after generation.

THE ECONOMIC TRAP: WHEN SURVIVAL TRUMPS SELF-CARE

You can't worry about eating healthy when you're choosing between groceries and rent. You can't prioritize checkups when taking a day off work might cost you your job, and you certainly can't afford prescriptions when your paycheck barely covers your light bill.

In Gary, Indiana, where I started my career, I saw firsthand how economic instability bleeds into every health decision. People e.g., steel mill workers, home health aides, warehouse staff working hard, living with chronic pain, untreated illnesses, and no plan for prevention. They weren't irresponsible. They were overworked, underpaid, and trying to make it through the week.

Economic barriers to healthcare literacy work in multiple ways. First, there's the obvious issue of access. When you can't afford to see a doctor regularly, you miss opportunities to learn about your health. You don't get the explanations, the printed materials, the follow-up conversations that help build understanding over time.

But the economic impact goes deeper than just affording appointments. When you're working multiple jobs to make ends meet, when do you have time to research your symptoms or read about your condition? When you're stressed about paying bills, how much mental energy do you have left to navigate insurance forms or understand treatment options?

Poverty also affects where you live, and where you live affects what healthcare resources are available. Community health centers in low-income areas often operate with skeleton staff, rushing patients through appointments. Pharmacies in these neighborhoods may not stock certain medications or offer counseling services. Even internet access which is crucial for health information is less reliable and more expensive in low-income communities.

The cruel irony is that the communities with the least economic resources often have the highest rates of chronic diseases that require the most health literacy to manage. Diabetes, hypertension, heart disease, kidney failure, these conditions demand daily attention, regular monitoring, and complex treatment regimens yet they disproportionately affect people who have the least support for understanding and managing them.

MEDICAL RACISM: WHEN THE SYSTEM SPEAKS IN CODE

Even when Black people make it into the healthcare system, the playing field is far from level. Medical racism isn't always loud. It's in the assumptions that patients won't follow up. In judgment when someone asks too many questions. In disbelief when a Black woman says, "I'm in pain."

I've been in the room when doctors changed their tone after I introduced myself as a nurse. Suddenly, they explained things better. Slowed down. Gave options. But before that? The patient, usually a Black patient, was talked at, not with.

This kind of treatment doesn't just hurt at the moment, it creates lasting damage to health literacy. When healthcare providers don't take time to explain conditions clearly, when they use medical jargon without checking for understanding, when they dismiss questions or concerns, patients leave appointments more confused than when they arrived.

Medical racism also shows up in the assumption that Black patients won't comply with treatment plans which contributes to the documenting and use of bias language. Instead of taking time to ensure understanding, providers might oversimplify instructions or skip explanations altogether. They might assume that complex treatment regimens are "too complicated" for certain patients, leading to inadequate care and poor outcomes.

The communication barriers are real. When providers don't look like you, don't come from your community, and don't understand your cultural context, the exchange of information becomes more difficult. Medical terms that might be clearly explained to white patients get rushed through with Black patients. Questions that would be welcomed from some are seen as challenging or difficult from others.

These experiences teach Black patients to be passive in medical encounters. If asking questions gets you labeled as difficult, if expressing concerns gets you dismissed, if advocating for yourself is seen as problematic, you learn to nod and smile and hope for the best. But passive patients are uninformed patients, and uninformed patients make poor health decisions.

WHEN MISINFORMATION FILLS THE VOID

When official systems fail, people turn to what they know: family, friends, and community. What happens when those trusted voices are misinformed?

Misinformation spreads where truth is missing. When doctors rush, when clinics close early, when language barriers go unaddressed, the vacuum gets filled with TikTok videos, Facebook posts, and well-meaning relatives who just want to help but don't have the right facts.

We can't blame people for listening to the voices that actually speak to them, especially when those voices look like them, sound like them, and come with no judgment. The consequences can be deadly when that information is wrong.

Social media has amplified this problem exponentially. Health misinformation spreads faster and reaches more people than ever before. Conspiracy theories about medical experimentation prey on legitimate historical concerns. Miracle cures and quick fixes appeal to people who can't afford traditional medical care. Anti-vaccine messages exploit fears about side effects while downplaying the risks of preventable diseases.

The community sources that people trust e.g., beauty salons, barbershops, churches, family gatherings become places where misinformation circulates alongside genuine care and concern. The challenge is that the same cultural networks that spread misinformation are also sources of genuine support and wisdom. These are the places where people feel heard, understood, and cared for.

The solution isn't to cut people off from their communities, it's to find ways to inject accurate health information into those trusted spaces.

THE FRAMEWORK THAT EXPLAINS IT ALL: SOCIAL DETERMINANTS OF HEALTH (SDOH)

All of these barriers we've discussed aren't random, they fit into a framework that public health experts call Social Determinants of Health. These are the conditions in which people live, learn, work, play and age that affect their health outcomes. There are five key domains, and understanding them helps explain why health literacy is so challenging in our communities.

Domain 1: Economic Stability

This goes beyond just having a job. Economic stability includes steady employment, living wages, manageable expenses, and protection from medical debt. When you're economically unstable, every health decision becomes a financial calculation. Can you afford to miss work for a doctor's appointment? Can you fill that prescription or pay your rent? Can you buy healthy food or keep the lights on?

Economic instability directly impacts health literacy because learning about your health requires time, mental energy, and often money, resources that are scarce when you're struggling financially. You might understand that exercise and healthy eating are important, but if you're working two jobs and living in a food desert, that knowledge doesn't translate into action.

Domain 2: Education Access and Quality

We've talked about how schools in our communities often fail to provide adequate health education. But this domain covers more than just health class. It includes early childhood education, literacy levels, language skills, and access to higher education.

When educational systems fail our communities, they create adults who may struggle to read medication labels, understand insurance forms, or research health conditions online. The literacy skills needed for general education are the same ones needed for health literacy. If the foundation is weak, everything else becomes harder.

Domain 3: Healthcare Access and Quality

This includes not just whether you can get healthcare, but whether that healthcare is high-quality, culturally competent, and accessible. It covers insurance coverage, provider availability, transportation to care, and whether services are offered in your language.

In our communities, we often face what's called "healthcare deserts", areas with limited access to primary care, specialists, or even pharmacies. When healthcare is hard to access or of poor quality, people miss opportunities to learn about their health, build relationships with providers, and develop the literacy skills needed for self-care.

Domain 4: Neighborhood and Built Environment

This is about where you live: housing quality, transportation options, walkability, access to healthy food, exposure to toxins, and neighborhood safety. Your environment shapes your health in ways you might not even realize.

If you live in a neighborhood without safe places to exercise, grocery stores with fresh produce, or reliable public transportation to medical appointments, your health options are limited before you even make a choice. Environmental stressors like pollution, noise, or violence also affect your ability to focus on health management and learning.

Domain 5: Social and Community Context

This includes social support, community cohesion, civic participation, workplace policies, and experiences with discrimination. It's about the social fabric that either supports or undermines your health.

In our communities, this domain is particularly complex. We have strong traditions of mutual support and community care, but we also face systemic discrimination that erodes trust in institutions. Historical trauma affects how communities share and receive health information. Social networks can either spread accurate health information or dangerous misinformation.

HOW THESE DETERMINANTS STEAL HEALTH LITERACY

Here's the crucial point: these five domains don't just affect your health, they affect your ability to understand and manage your health. Poor social determinants create what researchers call "cognitive load", when you're constantly dealing with stress from unstable housing, food insecurity, discrimination, or economic pressure, you have less mental energy available for processing health information.

Think about it this way: if you're worried about keeping your job, finding safe childcare, or avoiding eviction, how much mental space do you have left to research your diabetes management or understand your insurance benefits? If you live in a neighborhood where the nearest pharmacy is an hour away and you don't have reliable transportation, how likely are you to ask detailed questions about your medications?

The social determinants create a web of barriers that make health literacy exponentially more difficult. Each barrier feeds into the others. Poor education limits economic opportunities. Economic instability affects housing options. Poor housing affects health outcomes. Poor health affects employment. The cycle continues, trapping families and communities in patterns that undermine both health and health literacy.

THE INTERSECTION OF ALL BARRIERS

These barriers don't exist in isolation, they compound and reinforce each other. Poor education combines with economic constraints to limit options. Medical racism intersects with historical trauma to erode trust. Misinformation flourishes where official sources have failed to provide clear, culturally relevant information.

Consider a single mother working two jobs, who never learned about preventive care in school, can't afford regular doctor visits, has had dismissive experiences with healthcare providers, and turns to social media for health advice. Each barrier makes the others worse. Each missed opportunity for health literacy creates more vulnerability to the next barrier.

This intersection explains why individual solutions like telling people to "just ask more questions" or "do more research" fall short. The barriers are systemic, which means the solutions need to be systemic too.

BREAKING DOWN THE BARRIERS

Understanding these barriers isn't meant to make you feel hopeless, it's meant to help you see the whole picture. Healthcare literacy doesn't exist in isolation. It's shaped by what we learn, what we can afford, how we're treated, and who we trust.

The darkness surrounding our health decisions didn't appear overnight. It was built, layer by layer, by systems designed without us in mind. Here's the good news: what was built can be broken down. What's hidden can be brought into the light.

Recognizing these barriers and understanding how they fit into the larger framework of social determinants is the first step to navigating around them. When you understand that your struggles with healthcare aren't personal failures but system failures, you can approach them differently. You can seek out alternative sources of education, find providers who respect your intelligence, connect with community resources that share accurate information.

You can also become part of the solution. When you gain health literacy skills, you can share them with family and friends. When you find providers who treat you with respect, you can recommend them to others. When you encounter misinformation in your community, you can gently correct it with facts.

The systemic barriers that keep Black communities in the dark about healthcare are real and powerful but they're not permanent. Every person who breaks through these barriers, who gains the knowledge and skills to navigate the healthcare system successfully, creates a crack in the wall that others can follow.

Your health literacy journey isn't just about you, it's about your family, your community, and future generations. The barriers were designed to keep us sick, confused, and dependent. We can design our own pathways to health, knowledge, and empowerment.

The light is there. The knowledge exists. The tools are available. The question is whether you're ready to reach for them, despite the barriers that were built to keep them from you.

Those lost years we talked about in Chapter 1? Many of them are stolen not by individual choices, but by systemic barriers that make healthy choices harder. Understanding those barriers and how they fit into the broader framework of social determinants is the first step to reclaiming what's rightfully yours: a long, healthy life built on knowledge, advocacy, and community support.

CHAPTER 4

The Deadly Delay – Why Black Patients Get Diagnosed Late

How many times have you heard someone in your family say, "I don't want to go to the doctor because I'm afraid of what they might find"? How many times have you put off that appointment, ignored that symptom, or convinced yourself that what you're feeling will probably go away on its own?

You're not alone in this thinking, but here's the hard truth: by the time many Black patients finally get diagnosed with serious conditions, it's often too late for the best treatment options. We're more likely to be diagnosed with cancer at later stages, diabetes after complications have set in, and heart disease after heart attacks have already occurred.

This isn't happening because we're careless or because we don't care about our health. It's happening because of a complex web of barriers such as healthcare literacy gaps, medical bias, economic constraints, and deep-rooted mistrust that create deadly delays between the first signs of illness and accurate diagnosis.

These delays are stealing years from our lives, and it's time we understood exactly how and why this happens, so we can fight back against it.

WHEN SUBTLE CHANGES GO UNNOTICED

Delayed diagnosis doesn't always look like someone ignoring obvious symptoms. Sometimes it looks like subtle changes that go unnoticed until the situation becomes dangerous. In Black families, where elders are often fiercely independent and deeply respected, those changes can be even harder to confront.

I once worked with a family whose matriarch, lovingly called Big Ma by her grandchildren and Ma'dea by her sons, had spent over 30 years working physically demanding jobs in the steel mills of Gary, Indiana. She was a single mother who raised two sons, retired, and lived independently in a senior living apartment. She had never learned to read or write, but she was proud, self-sufficient, and closely connected to her family.

Over time, she began showing signs of confusion. The changes were subtle. So subtle that her sons and great-niece, who saw her often, did not notice. It was her granddaughter who first raised concerns, but denial kept the family from acting on them. What no one realized at the time was that these were early signs of Alzheimer's Disease.

One night, her son called his daughter in a panic because Ma'Dea was not answering her phone and he was afraid to enter her apartment. The family rushed over and discovered she was gone. Checking her answering machine, they later learned she had been taken from her senior apartment complex by healthcare staff and transported across state lines to a hospital in Illinois.

She had been admitted with a chief complaint of bradycardia, a low heart rate. When the family arrived, she had no idea she had even been taken. She thought they were just visiting. The family confronted hospital staff, questioned the legitimacy of the admission, and demanded her discharge. Shortly after, she was released.

This situation revealed something much deeper than a heart issue. It exposed how vulnerable, elderly, academically illiterate and health illiterate patients can be taken advantage of, especially when they live alone and are trying to protect their independence.

Big Ma's story illustrates a critical point: when early cognitive decline is missed, patients are at greater risk for being mismanaged, misunderstood, and in some cases, scammed. This is how deadly delays happen. Not always through neglect, but through lack of awareness and lack of protection.

WHEN MENTAL HEALTH LABELS MASK PHYSICAL ILLNESS

Sometimes the delay in diagnosis happens because healthcare providers see one condition and miss another. This is especially dangerous when mental health issues become labels that prevent proper investigation of physical symptoms.

I worked with a woman known as "Queen" to her friends, a Black woman in her 50s who struggled with mental illness. She visited her local ER, primary care doctor, and mental health providers both scheduled and unscheduled, and by some accounts was labeled as a "frequent flier" defined as someone who treats the emergency room like a doctor's office instead of using it only for urgent issues.

During the Winter Season, she exhibited signs of Seasonal Affective Disorder (SAD) in combination with Depression. SAD describes people who do very well in the Summer months when daylight is extended but become reclusive and homebound during the Winter, when it's cold and daylight hours are shorter. Her mental health signs and symptoms meant that she would have days where she was overly excited, demonstrated impulsive and hoarding-type buying, and down days where she just wanted to go to bed and cover her head.

Even though she went to the ER for everything, even minor illnesses that should have been handled by her primary care doctor, she did have a serious health issue brewing inside her, one that went undiagnosed for some time. One day, she shared with her sibling that she was urinating a lot and she even experienced excessive vaginal bleeding though she was post-menopausal. Her sister urged her to see a gynecologist and a urologist.

When she finally secured these appointments, following one of her frequent ER visits, she was diagnosed with renal carcinoma or cancer of the kidney. The initial surgical procedure was for a partial nephrectomy (removal of a piece of a kidney), which later resulted in a total nephrectomy (removal of the entire kidney).

Queen's story shows how patients with healthcare literacy challenges struggle to adequately describe their signs and symptoms, or they omit telling the healthcare team things because they assume one thing has nothing to do with the other. The result is a work-up based on what the patient reported, not what they didn't report. With early intervention, some or all of the kidney may have been saved.

THE PERFECT STORM OF DELAYED DIAGNOSIS

These stories aren't isolated incidents. They represent patterns that play out in Black communities across the country, where multiple factors combine to create dangerous delays in diagnosis:

The Screening Gap

We simply don't get screened as often or as early as we should. Part of this is access. If you don't have insurance or a regular doctor, preventive screenings fall by the wayside. Part of it is education. If no one ever explained that colonoscopies start at age 45 for Black Americans, or that mammograms should begin at 40, how would you know? Part of it is trust. If you're not sure the medical system has your best interests at heart, you're less likely to seek care before you feel sick.

The result is that conditions that could be caught early through routine screening like colon cancer, breast cancer, cervical cancer, diabetes, chronic kidney disease, hypertension often aren't diagnosed until symptoms appear. By then, treatment is more difficult, more expensive, and less likely to be successful.

The Communication Breakdown

When we do see healthcare providers, communication problems often prevent accurate and timely diagnosis. If you can't clearly describe your symptoms because you lack the medical vocabulary, providers might miss important clues. If you don't understand what questions the doctor is asking, you might not give complete answers. If cultural differences create barriers to open communication, crucial information doesn't get shared.

Queen's experience illustrates this perfectly. She was in the healthcare system constantly, but her mental health label overshadowed her physical symptoms. Her difficulty communicating the connection between her urinary changes and other symptoms delayed proper investigation. When patients can't advocate effectively for themselves, important signs get missed.

The Bias Factor

Medical bias plays a huge role in delayed diagnosis for Black patients. Our pain gets taken less seriously. Our symptoms are more likely to be attributed to lifestyle factors. Our concerns are more easily dismissed. Research consistently shows that Black patients receive different quality of care, and this directly affects how quickly and accurately we get diagnosed.

When Queen was labeled a "frequent flier," healthcare providers began seeing her through that lens rather than taking each visit seriously. When Big Ma was vulnerable due to cognitive decline, the system saw an opportunity for exploitation rather than a need for protection. These biases create blind spots that can be literally deadly.

The Trust Deficit

The historical betrayals we discussed in Chapter 2 create ongoing reluctance to seek medical care. If you don't trust the system, you're more likely to tough out symptoms, rely on home remedies, or seek help only when conditions become undeniable. By then, what could have been treated easily becomes a medical emergency.

This mistrust also affects how honestly patients communicate with providers. If you're not sure you can trust your doctor, you might not mention embarrassing symptoms, you might downplay the severity of your pain, or you might not follow up when something doesn't feel right.

THE CASCADE EFFECT OF LATE DIAGNOSIS

When diagnosis is delayed, everything that follows becomes more difficult and more dangerous. Early-stage cancers that are 90% curable become advanced cancers with survival rates below 20%. Diabetes that could be managed with lifestyle changes becomes diabetes requiring insulin and monitoring for complications. High blood pressure that could be controlled with one medication becomes hypertensive crisis requiring multiple drugs and emergency intervention. Chronic Kidney Disease that could be managed with mediation becomes End Stage Renal Disease requiring dialysis three times a week.

Late diagnosis doesn't just affect the individual, it affects families, communities, and the next generation. Children who watch their parents suffer from preventable complications learn to fear and avoid healthcare. Families that lose primary breadwinners to diseases that could have been caught early face economic devastation. Communities lose elders, leaders, and knowledge holders to conditions that modern medicine knows how to treat.

This is how the "lost decade" happens. Not all at once, but year by year, delay by delay, missed opportunity by missed opportunity. Each late diagnosis represents not just individual suffering, but collective loss.

RECOGNIZING THE WARNING SIGNS

Part of preventing delayed diagnosis is learning to recognize when subtle changes might signal serious health problems. If you notice a loved one becoming increasingly forgetful, missing meals, getting lost in familiar places, or struggling with daily routines, these may be early signs of dementia or Alzheimer's Disease. The earlier these changes are recognized, the more options families have to protect their loved one's safety and dignity.

Similarly, physical symptoms that persist, worsen, or seem unusual deserve medical attention, even if they seem minor. Frequent urination, unexplained bleeding, persistent pain, changes in appetite or weight, or new lumps or bumps should all prompt medical evaluation.

The key is not waiting until symptoms become severe or until you "can't take it anymore." Early intervention almost always means better outcomes, more treatment options, and less invasive procedures.

BREAKING THE CYCLE OF DELAY

Preventing delayed diagnosis requires action on multiple levels. Healthcare systems need to address bias in training and practice. Communities need better access to preventive care and health education. Families need to develop health literacy skills that help them recognize concerning symptoms and advocate effectively for care.

But while we're working on these systemic changes, there are steps you can take right now to protect yourself and your family:

Build relationships with healthcare providers before you get sick. Having an established relationship with a primary care provider makes it easier to get timely appointments and honest communication when concerns arise.

Learn your family health history and share it. Understanding what conditions run in your family helps you and your providers know what to watch for and when to start screening.

Keep track of symptoms and changes. Write down when symptoms started, what makes them better or worse, and how they're affecting your daily life. This information helps providers make more accurate diagnoses.

Ask questions and seek clarification. Don't leave medical appointments confused. Make sure you understand your diagnosis, treatment plan, and what symptoms should prompt immediate medical attention.

Get second opinions for serious diagnoses. Different providers may see things differently or have different treatment approaches. Getting another perspective can help ensure you're getting the best care.

Trust your instincts. If something doesn't feel right, even if others dismiss your concerns, seek medical attention. You know your body better than anyone else.

THE PROMISE OF EARLY DETECTION

When Black patients do receive timely, appropriate care, outcomes improve dramatically. Early-stage breast cancer has a five-year survival rate above 98%. Colon cancer caught through screening is often completely preventable through polyp removal. Diabetes identified early can often be managed through lifestyle changes alone.

The technology and knowledge exist to catch most serious conditions early when they're most treatable. The challenge is making sure that Black communities have equal access to this early detection and that our symptoms are taken seriously when we seek care.

UNDERSTANDING THE SILENT THREAT

These delayed diagnoses aren't happening with rare, exotic diseases. They're happening with common conditions that kill Black Americans at disproportionate rates, conditions that could be prevented or caught early if we knew what to look for and when to look for it.

The conditions that most often go undiagnosed in our communities aren't random. They're what medical professionals call "silent killers", diseases that develop quietly, without obvious symptoms, until they reach dangerous or even fatal stages. Hypertension earned its nickname "the silent killer." Diabetes silently damages organs for years before symptoms appear. Certain cancers grow undetected until they've spread and chronic kidney disease damages the kidneys' resulting in kidney failure.

Big Ma's cognitive changes were subtle and silent until they became dangerous. Queen's kidney cancer developed without obvious early symptoms, hidden behind her mental health challenges. Most preventable killers in our communities share this silent nature, which makes understanding them crucial for protecting yourself and your family.

Every delayed diagnosis represents a missed opportunity, not just for that individual, but for their family and community. Every early diagnosis represents hope, longer life, and the possibility that we can start to close the gap in health outcomes that has persisted for far too long.

The "lost decade" doesn't have to be permanent. With better health literacy, stronger advocacy skills, improved access to care, and systemic changes to address bias and barriers, we can catch conditions early and treat them effectively.

Your health is too important to leave to chance, and your life is too valuable to lose to preventable delays. The goal isn't just to live longer, it's to live better, with the knowledge, skills, and support needed to catch problems early and address them effectively.

Understanding delayed diagnosis is just the first step. The next step is recognizing which specific conditions are most likely to slip past our defenses and why they're so deadly when we finally discover them. Because when you know what the silent killers look like, you're better equipped to catch them before they can steal those precious years from your life.

TIPS FROM DR. CARLA'S CARING CORNER

- If you notice your loved one is becoming forgetful more than a few times a day, stops eating or taking meds, gets confused or lost in the grocery store where they shopped for years, drives some place but can't remember how to get back home, clothes don't match…this could be the early signs of Dementia, one of which is Alzheimer's.
- Talk to a doctor such as a neurologist for brain changes and psychiatrist or psychologist for the behavioral changes noted. As the disease progresses, you will need to see other healthcare providers depending on what part of the body or system is affected by the disease.
- Medicare rules say patients being considered for a nursing home or similar housing must be hospitalized for 72 hours. Discharge planning by a social worker or discharge planner will take this into consideration should your loved one need more care immediately after the hospitalization is over. It is easier to transition them directly from the hospital than to take them home first.

- A senior center is not the same as assisted living. Assisted living indicates there are additional services (emphasis on assisted) such as healthcare and even laundry services for a higher fee.
- If your loved one is in a senior living center, inquire as to what health & wellness takes place. What are some examples the facility would call the emergency contact for. Above all, check in routinely on your loved ones and attend their doctor's visits with them even if they feel like you are babying them.

(TIPS FROM SECOND STORY)

- Doctoral prepared registered nurses are a wealth of information and can deliver patient/disease-specific education and training to individuals and organizations.
- Always inform healthcare providers when you have undergone major surgery like the removal of a kidney so they prescribe medications/treatments that are renal-protective, meaning medication that does not further damage your only existing kidney.
- Adopt lifestyle changes that protect your organs like a kidney so that you minimize the possibility of being on dialysis for the rest of your life which is a three-day a week regimen for people with end stage renal disease (ESRD) also inherent to Blacks.

CHAPTER 5

Silent Killers – Common but Preventable Causes of Early Death

Do you know what's killing us? I don't mean the obvious dangers e.g., the violence that makes headlines, the accidents that seem random, the rare diseases that get all the research funding. I'm talking about the quiet killers, the ones that move through our communities like shadows, taking our fathers, mothers, siblings, and friends years before their time.

These silent killers have names you know well: heart disease, stroke, diabetes, high blood pressure, kidney disease. They're called "silent" not because they don't make noise when they finally strike, but because they work quietly for years, decades even, without obvious symptoms. By the time you feel them, by the time they force you to pay attention, they've often done irreversible damage.

Here's what makes this tragedy even worse: most of these killers are preventable. The conditions that are stealing a decade of life from Black Americans are largely diseases we know how to prevent, treat, and manage. Yet they continue to devastate our communities at rates that should make everyone angry.

The question isn't whether these diseases exist, they do, and they're not going anywhere. The question is whether you're going to let them catch you unprepared, or whether you're going to arm yourself with the knowledge and tools to fight back.

WHEN THE HEART STOPS TALKING

Heart disease is the number one killer of Black Americans, and it's particularly deadly for Black men. But here's what's frustrating: the signs are often there long before the heart attack, the sudden cardiac death, or the need for emergency surgery. The problem is that these signs often speak in a language we haven't learned to understand.

Arthur, a 60-year-old Black man, dedicated his career to the military both at home and abroad. He even relocated for greater upward mobility and wasn't concerned about insurance coverage. He believed in healthcare as a lifelong military man. While on a trip stateside, he went to the doctor for a cardiac workup. When he left the office, he wasn't quite sure what to make of the many calls and texts he received from the facility. He even felt their incessant calls had started to annoy him and become downright intrusive. Fortunately, he eventually called them back.

What they told him was that he had an abnormally low heart rate in the 40s (normal is 60-100 bpm) and that he had an arrhythmia known as third-degree heart block. He wasn't sure what it meant, but he recalls always living with a low heart rate. Third-degree heart block is the deadliest rhythm of the heart blocks because the electrical signals between the heart chambers are blocked. When this occurs, blood flow is compromised. They informed him that the treatment for this problem was to undergo insertion of an automated internal cardiac defibrillator (AICD) and that a delay could result in his untimely death.

The question that haunts Arthur's story is: Why wasn't this deadly rhythm diagnosed earlier in his military career? How many physicals, how many routine checkups, how many opportunities were there to catch this condition before it became life-threatening?

Arthur's experience illustrates a critical point about silent killers: they're often not as silent as we think. The signs are there, the low heart rate he'd always lived with, the subtle symptoms that might have been dismissed as normal aging or stress. Without health literacy, without understanding what these signs mean and when they require immediate action, we miss opportunities for early intervention.

WHEN PRIDE BECOMES DEADLY

Sometimes the silent killer isn't the disease itself, it's the shame, fear, or pride that prevents us from seeking proper treatment. This is particularly true for Black men, who face unique challenges when it comes to managing conditions like hypertension.

"Lil Bro" affectionately known to his friends, a 60-year-old Black man who spent his life working in the steel mills of East Chicago, Indiana. He was divorced, lived alone, was estranged from his children, but did enjoy a full life with friends. He smoked, consumed his fair share of alcohol and remained sexually active with the help of medications like Viagra and Cialis. What he did not realize was that he had a heart problem.

Once his heart disease was diagnosed, the recommendation was for him to undergo a coronary artery bypass graft (CABG), a surgery where the chest is cracked and held open with rib spreaders while surgeons work to redirect blood flow away from damaged blood vessels. After surgery, patients are placed in the intensive care unit on a ventilator, hopefully for a short time.

But here's the critical piece of Lil Bro's story: men who take medications like nitrates aka Nitroglycerin for chest pain, phosphodiesterase type 5 (PDE5) for Erectile Dysfunction (ED) or sexual problems, anti-hypertensives to lower blood pressure, smoke and/or consume alcohol are at risk of experiencing cardiac events and should refrain from taking medications that help with Erectile Dysfunction. Hypertension is common among African Americans and is attributed to factors like heredity, diet, and other lifestyle factors. Black men are often hesitant to take the medication required to treat hypertension because a common side effect is Erectile Dysfunction.

Black men are already predisposed to diseases like stroke, but many are more consumed with their sex life or feelings of sexual inadequacy than with life itself. Instead of taking life-saving medications, they choose to skip, omit, or otherwise avoid taking their blood pressure medications.

I followed Lil Bro's care as best I could, accompanied him to his doctor's visits, and even completed his disability paperwork so he could retire from the mills. Surgery and timely retirement got him a few more years, but he still died on a ventilator in an ICU a decade sooner than he should have.

This isn't just an individual problem, it's a community health crisis. Even in prisons, where you might think men would prioritize their health, incarcerated men engaging in sexual activity refuse their blood pressure medications for the same reason men on the outside do: fear of ED. Incarcerated patients who don't take their blood pressure medications can experience hypertension, kidney failure, diabetes, heart disease, stroke, and more making this a national imperative as, upon release, their communities will absorb their medical problems.

THE BIG THREE: OUR COMMUNITY'S SILENT ASSASSINS

While there are many conditions that disproportionately affect Black Americans, three stand out as the deadliest and most preventable:

Hypertension: The True Silent Killer

High blood pressure affects nearly 60% of Black adults. Almost double the rate of white Americans. It's called the silent killer because it often has no symptoms until it causes a heart attack, stroke, or kidney failure. Your blood pressure can be dangerously high for years while you feel perfectly fine.

What makes hypertension particularly deadly in our communities isn't just the higher rates, it's the poor control rates. Even when Black Americans are diagnosed with high blood pressure, we're less likely to have it properly managed. This leads to more heart attacks, more strokes, more kidney disease, and more early deaths.

The barriers to proper hypertension management include medication side effects (like the erectile dysfunction that kept Lil Bro from taking his pills), medication costs, lack of understanding about the seriousness of the condition, and mistrust of the healthcare system.

Diabetes: The Slow Destroyer

Type 2 diabetes affects Black Americans at nearly twice the rate of white Americans, and we're more likely to develop serious complications. Diabetes is particularly insidious because it can damage your kidneys, eyes, nerves, and blood vessels for years before you notice symptoms.

By the time many Black Americans are diagnosed with diabetes, they already have complications that could have been prevented with earlier detection and proper management. Poor health literacy plays a huge role here if you don't understand how diabetes works, if you don't know what blood sugar numbers mean, if you don't understand the connection between diet and blood sugar, you can't effectively manage the condition.

Heart Disease: The Number One Killer

Heart disease kills more Black Americans than any other condition, and we're more likely to die from it at younger ages. Like Arthur's story shows, heart problems often develop over years or decades, with warning signs that go unrecognized or ignored.

The challenge with heart disease is that it requires understanding multiple risk factors and how they interact. High blood pressure, diabetes, high cholesterol, smoking, obesity, and family history all contribute to heart disease risk. Without health literacy, it's hard to understand how all these pieces fit together and what you can do to lower your risk.

WHY WE'RE HIT HARDER

The disproportionate impact of these silent killers on Black communities isn't accidental or inevitable. It's the result of multiple factors working together to create perfect storms for poor health outcomes:

Environmental Factors

Where you live affects your health in ways you might not even realize. Many Black communities are located in areas with higher pollution levels, fewer safe spaces for exercise, limited access to healthy food, and higher levels of chronic stress. These environmental factors contribute to higher rates of hypertension, diabetes, and heart disease.

Food deserts, areas without access to affordable, nutritious food, make it nearly impossible to follow the dietary recommendations that could prevent or manage these conditions. When the closest grocery store is miles away but there's a fast-food restaurant on every corner, healthy eating becomes a luxury rather than a realistic option.

Economic Barriers

The cost of managing chronic conditions can be overwhelming. Monthly medications, regular doctor visits, blood tests, and lifestyle changes all require financial resources that many families simply don't have. When you're choosing between medications and rent, between healthy food and utility bills, health often loses.

The cruel irony is that preventing these conditions is much less expensive than treating their complications, but the healthcare system is set up to pay for treatment rather than prevention. Insurance will cover dialysis for kidney failure but not always the nutritionist who could help prevent diabetes complications.

Healthcare Quality Disparities

Even when Black Americans do access healthcare, we often receive lower-quality care. We're less likely to receive optimal medications for heart conditions, less likely to be referred to specialists when needed, and more likely to have our pain and concerns dismissed.

These quality disparities mean that even when we're in the healthcare system, we're not getting the full benefit of what modern medicine has to offer. Conditions that could be well-controlled with proper treatment become poorly managed, leading to complications and early death.

BREAKING THE SILENCE

The good news is that silent killers lose their power when you know how to recognize and fight them. Here's what you need to know to protect yourself and your family:

Know Your Numbers

You can't manage what you don't measure. Every Black adult should know their:

- Blood pressure (goal: less than 130/80)
- Blood sugar (fasting glucose less than 100)
- Cholesterol levels (LDL less than 100)
- Body mass index (BMI 18.5-24.9)
- Family history of chronic diseases

Understand the Connections

These conditions don't exist in isolation. High blood pressure increases your risk of heart disease and stroke. Diabetes increases your risk of kidney disease and heart disease. Obesity increases your risk of diabetes and high blood pressure. Understanding these connections helps you see why managing one condition helps prevent others.

Get Past the Shame and Fear

Lil Bro's story shows how shame about medication side effects can literally kill you. If you're experiencing side effects from medications, talk to your healthcare provider about alternatives. There are many different blood pressure medications, and most men can find options that don't cause Erectile Dysfunction.

If you're worried about sexual function, remember that being dead eliminates all sexual function permanently. The goal is finding treatments that allow you to live a long, healthy life with good quality of life including sexual health.

Build Your Health Literacy

Learn what your conditions mean, how your medications work, and what lifestyle changes can help. Ask questions at every appointment. Bring a list or bag of your medications and know what each one does. Understand what symptoms require immediate medical attention.

COMMUNITY SOLUTIONS THAT WORK

While individual action is important, community-level solutions have shown the most promise for reducing the impact of these silent killers:

Community Health Workers

Programs that train community members to provide health education and support have been particularly successful in Black communities. These health workers understand the cultural context, speak the language of the community, and can provide ongoing support for managing chronic conditions.

Faith-Based Health Programs

Churches and other faith communities have natural networks for sharing health information and providing support. Programs that work through these existing structures have been successful in increasing blood pressure control, diabetes management, and healthy lifestyle adoption.

Workplace Wellness Programs

For communities like the steel workers that Lil Bro worked with, workplace wellness programs can reach men who might not otherwise seek healthcare. On-site screenings, health education, and support for medication management can catch problems early and improve outcomes.

Community Gardens and Food Programs

Addressing food access through community gardens, farmers' markets, and healthy food initiatives can make it easier for families to adopt the dietary changes that help prevent and manage these conditions.

THE FIGHT FOR MORE YEARS

Arthur and Lil Bro's stories represent thousands of Black men whose lives were and may be shortened by silent killers that could have been detected and managed earlier. Arthur's heart condition had probably been developing for years before it was finally caught. Lil Bro's heart disease was manageable, but his reluctance to take blood pressure medications and the system's failure to address his concerns about side effects cost him years of life.

These silent killers are stealing a decade of life from Black Americans, but they don't have to. With better health literacy, improved access to care, community support programs, and systemic changes to address the root causes of health disparities, we can fight back.

The conditions that kill us most often e.g., heart disease, stroke, diabetes, high blood pressure, kidney disease are largely preventable and manageable. The knowledge exists. The treatments work. The question is whether we'll develop the individual skills and community systems needed to identify these killers early and fight them effectively.

Your life is too valuable to lose to a preventable disease. Your family needs you to be healthy and present for as long as possible. Your community can't afford to keep losing people to conditions that we know how to treat.

The silent killers are only silent if you don't know what to listen for. Once you understand their language, the elevated blood pressure readings, the family history patterns, the gradual symptom changes you can hear them coming and take action to stop them.

Those ten years that healthcare disparities are stealing from our communities? Many of them are being taken by these silent killers. Armed with knowledge, supported by the community, and commitment to long-term health rather than short-term convenience, you can reclaim those years and help others do the same.

The fight against silent killers starts with breaking the silence, talking openly about these conditions, sharing information within families and communities, and refusing to accept that early death from preventable diseases is normal or inevitable.

It's not normal. It's not inevitable and with the right knowledge and support, it's not going to be your story.

TIPS FROM DR. CARLA'S CARING CORNER

- Signs and symptoms of 3rd Degree Heartblock are only discernable with certain tests.
- See a doctor if you experience faintness, increased tiredness or shortness of breath.
- Athletes routinely have low heart rates. This does not mean they have a heart block. It means their bodies have learned to live with lower rates because they are so active and experience increased cardiac work out.

- Heart blocks contribute to the disease known as congestive heart failure and compromises your overall cardiac function.

- Medication prescribed to help your heart and AICD to function optimally should never be discontinued without provider approval.

[From Second Story]

- Significant others e.g. wives, girlfriends, friends-with-benefits to men on anti-hypertensives should support them in finding alternative methods of intimacy as an alternative to intercourse.

- Seek medical help for ED but never discontinue prescribed medication. Even though you may stop taking your meds, the disease process does not take a break from silently stealing decades of your life.

- A Penile implant is a surgical procedure that helps extend a man's erection for periods of time. It has pros/cons but certainly worth investigating. Consult with a Urologist or surgeon for this and other alternative treatments for Erectile Dysfunction.

- Hypertension(HTN) is the disease known as the silent killer. The symptoms are so subtle that most people ignore them. It ravages the body and the blood vessels while sending very subtle and silent signals e.g., headache, or nausea that can be easily ignored or treated with over-the-counter medication e.g. acetaminophen or drinking clear carbonated beverages like Sprite or 7-Up.

One common result of untreated Hypertension(HTN) is Stroke either thrombotic or hemorrhagic meaning a blood clot that just sits in one place like a snowball getting bigger until blood can no longer get around it, or one where it gets tired of sitting around and growing so it breaks away and travels. Common areas of travel are the lungs or the brain, both of which can kill you. One never knows the severity or magnitude of the signs/symptoms until they experience a massive stroke and present in the emergency room or morgue and never knew what hit them.

CHAPTER 6

The Emergency Room is Not a Doctor's Office

At 2 AM on any given Tuesday, walk into the emergency room of a hospital serving a Black community, and you'll see what America's healthcare crisis looks like up close. A grandmother holding a crying baby with an ear infection that's been building for three days. A man in work clothes clutching his chest, unsure if it's heartburn or something worse. A woman who ran out of blood pressure medication last week and is scared to wait until Monday to see if she can get an appointment. A father trying to get a sports physical for his son to play basketball.

This scene plays out every night in emergency rooms across America. People who aren't having medical emergencies sitting alongside people who are dying, all waiting for care in the one place that's always open, always available, and required by law to see them regardless of their ability to pay.

But here's what we need to understand: the emergency room is designed for emergencies. When we use it as our doctor's office, everyone suffers, the true emergency patients who have to wait longer, the hospitals that get overwhelmed and have to go on bypass, the healthcare system that becomes less efficient, and us, because we're not getting the right kind of care for our needs.

The overuse of emergency rooms isn't just inconvenient or expensive, it's contributing to the decade of life we're losing. It delays proper diagnosis, prevents effective management of chronic conditions, creates crushing medical debt, and keeps us from building the ongoing relationships with healthcare providers that could save our lives.

Understanding when to use the ER and when to seek other care isn't just about being a good healthcare consumer, it's about protecting your health, your finances, and your future.

WHY THE ER BECAME OUR DOCTOR

The relationship between Black communities and emergency rooms didn't develop overnight. It's the result of decades of healthcare policies, economic realities, and systemic barriers that pushed people toward emergency care as their only reliable option.

When Primary Care Isn't Available

In many Black communities, finding a primary care doctor feels impossible. Clinics close early, appointments are booked weeks out, providers don't take your insurance e.g. Medicaid/MediCal, or there simply aren't enough doctors in your neighborhood. When you're sick and need care, the emergency room becomes the only place that's open, available, and required by law to see you regardless of your ability to pay.

This creates a cycle: because people use the ER for primary care, fewer primary care providers want to practice in these communities. Because there are fewer primary care providers, more people end up in the ER. The problem feeds itself while communities suffer.

The Trust Factor

After generations of poor treatment in traditional healthcare settings, some people find the ER feels safer. There are witnesses, other staff, other patients. You can't be easily dismissed or ignored when you're in a busy emergency room. The ER also operates under different rules like Emergency Medical Treatment and Labor Act (EMTALA) than private practices, with legal obligations to stabilize patients regardless of their insurance status or ability to pay.

For people who have experienced discrimination in doctors' offices, the ER can feel like a more neutral space where they're more likely to be heard and helped.

The 24/7 Reality

Health problems don't follow a 9-to-5 schedule, but most primary care practices do. When your blood pressure spikes on Saturday night, when your diabetes makes you feel dizzy on Sunday morning, when your child's fever climbs on a holiday, the ER is the only option that's always available.

For families managing multiple jobs, unpredictable schedules, and limited time off, the ER's round-the-clock availability can seem like the most practical option, even for non-emergency issues.

THE OTHER EXTREME: WHEN EMERGENCY CARE IS AVOIDED ENTIRELY

While many people overuse emergency rooms, there's another dangerous pattern in our communities: people who avoid medical care entirely, even when they desperately need emergency treatment. This avoidance can be just as deadly as overuse.

I once knew a woman named Kid Comer, a 60-year-old Black woman who lived alone, never married, and had no children. She was deeply devoted to her church and believed her faith alone was enough to protect her health. She often gave testimony about how old she was and how she had never been to the doctor.

She was morbidly obese and showed signs of both physical and behavioral health challenges, yet she proudly wore her "healthcare free" lifestyle as a badge of honor. She got nearly all of her information, including health information, from the church. Even when the Bible itself speaks of Luke as a physician, she rejected the idea that medical care had a place in her life.

When the Covid pandemic began, she, like most people, self-isolated, relying on her belief that she had lived a disease-free life. As she became ill, family and church members urged her to seek medical care, but she refused. Afraid of contracting Covid-19, they checked on her by telephone. As her health continued to decline, she refused pleas to go to the hospital.

Days later, she was found dead on her living room sofa.

Kid Comer's story represents the other extreme of the emergency room problem. While some people use the ER as their doctor's office, others avoid even emergency care when their lives depend on it. Both patterns, overuse and complete avoidance contribute to poor health outcomes in our communities.

This is what happens when the emergency room is viewed as either the only option or not an option at all. Faith is powerful. Community is powerful. Neither should replace medical care when it's truly needed. They are meant to work together, not against each other.

THE REAL COST OF GETTING IT WRONG

Using the emergency room inappropriately, whether that's going too often for minor issues or avoiding it when you truly need emergency care comes with serious consequences that extend far beyond the individual patient.

Financial Devastation

An emergency room visit can cost anywhere from $500 to $3,000 or more, depending on what tests and treatments you receive. The same care at an urgent care clinic might cost $150-300. A visit to your primary care doctor might cost $100-200. When you multiply these differences over time, families can face crushing medical debt for care that could have been provided much more affordably elsewhere.

I've seen families declare bankruptcy because of emergency room bills for conditions that could have been managed in a doctor's office. The financial stress of medical debt affects every aspect of life e.g., housing, education, employment opportunities and can perpetuate the very conditions that lead to poor health in the first place.

Delayed and Fragmented Care

Emergency rooms are designed to stabilize patients and send them home or admit them to the hospital. They're not designed to provide ongoing care for chronic conditions like diabetes, hypertension, or heart disease. When you use the ER as your primary care provider, you get fragmented care from different doctors who don't know your history and can't provide the continuity that chronic disease management requires.

This fragmentation leads to missed opportunities for prevention, poor medication management, and delayed diagnosis of serious conditions. You might get your blood pressure treated in the ER today, but if there's no follow-up, no medication adjustment, no lifestyle counseling, the underlying problem continues to worsen.

System Overload

When emergency rooms are overwhelmed with non-emergency cases, truly emergency patients people having heart attacks, strokes, or severe injuries have to wait longer for life-saving care. This affects everyone in the community and can literally mean the difference between life and death for people with true emergencies.

Healthcare workers in overloaded emergency rooms also suffer from burnout, which affects the quality of care they can provide. When nurses and doctors are overwhelmed and exhausted, everyone's care suffers.

Missed Prevention Opportunities

Perhaps most importantly, using the ER for primary care means missing out on the preventive services that could catch problems early. Emergency rooms don't do mammograms, colonoscopies, or routine blood work to screen for diabetes. They don't provide the health education, lifestyle counseling, and ongoing monitoring that prevent minor problems from becoming major crises. They exist to treat the single complaint that brought you to the ER.

When Kid Comer avoided all medical care, she missed decades of opportunities for blood pressure monitoring, diabetes screening, weight management support, and other services that might have helped her live longer and healthier. When people use only emergency care, they get some of these opportunities, but not the comprehensive, coordinated approach that produces the best health outcomes.

LEARNING TO NAVIGATE THE SYSTEM

The solution isn't to avoid the emergency room entirely or to use it for everything. The solution is learning when emergency care is truly needed and developing alternatives for other health concerns.

True Medical Emergencies

You should go to the emergency room immediately for:

- Chest pain or pressure, especially with shortness of breath, sweating, or nausea
- Signs of stroke: sudden weakness, numbness, confusion, trouble speaking, severe headache
- Severe difficulty breathing or shortness of breath
- Serious injuries or trauma
- Severe abdominal pain
- High fever with stiff neck, confusion, or rash

- Severe allergic reactions
- Thoughts of suicide or harming others
- Any condition where you feel your life is in immediate danger

Urgent but Not Emergency Care

For conditions that need attention within 24 hours but aren't life-threatening, consider urgent care clinics:

- Minor cuts that might need stitches
- Sprains and strains
- Fever without other serious symptoms
- Ear infections
- Urinary tract infections
- Minor burns
- Rashes or skin infections

Urgent care clinics are typically much less expensive than emergency rooms, have shorter wait times, and are specifically designed for these types of problems and always accept walk-ins.

Primary Care Issues

For ongoing health management and non-urgent concerns, work on establishing a relationship with a primary care provider:

- Routine checkups and screenings
- Management of chronic conditions like diabetes and high blood pressure
- Prescription refills
- Follow-up care after hospitalization, illness or injury

- Health education and prevention counseling
- Mental health support

Building Your Healthcare Team

Instead of relying on the emergency room for all your healthcare needs, work on building a team of providers who can address different aspects of your health:

Primary Care Provider: Your main doctor who coordinates your overall care and knows your health history.

Pharmacy: A trusted pharmacist who can answer medication questions and help manage drug interactions.

Community Health Center: Federally qualified health centers (FQHC) often provide affordable care on sliding fee scales.

Mental Health Support: Counselors, therapists, or spiritual advisors who can help with emotional and psychological health.

Specialists: When needed for specific conditions, accessed through referrals from your primary care provider.

COMMUNITY SOLUTIONS THAT WORK

Some communities have successfully reduced emergency room overuse while improving health outcomes through innovative programs and policy changes.

Community Health Workers

Programs that train community members to provide basic health education and help people navigate the healthcare system have been particularly effective in reducing unnecessary ER visits. These health workers can help people understand when different types of care are appropriate and how to access them.

Extended Hours Clinics

Community health centers that offer evening and weekend hours provide alternatives to emergency room care for people who can't take time off work during regular business hours.

Telehealth Services

Phone and video consultations can help people determine whether their symptoms require immediate emergency care, urgent care, or can wait for a regular appointment. This technology has been particularly helpful for mental health support and chronic disease management.

Faith Community Partnerships

Working with churches and other faith communities to provide health education has been effective in reaching people who might otherwise avoid medical care entirely. These programs can help people understand that faith and medical care can work together rather than in opposition.

Mobile Health Units

Bringing healthcare directly to underserved communities through mobile clinics helps provide preventive care and early intervention that reduces the need for emergency services.

FINDING THE BALANCE

Kid Comer's story reminds us that avoiding all medical care can be just as dangerous as overusing emergency services. The goal is finding the right balance using emergency care when it's truly needed, seeking appropriate alternatives for urgent but non-emergency issues, and building ongoing relationships with healthcare providers for prevention and chronic disease management.

This balance requires health literacy, understanding what different symptoms mean, knowing what types of care are available, and feeling confident advocating for yourself in various healthcare settings. It also requires access like having realistic options besides the emergency room when you need medical attention.

RECLAIMING THOSE LOST YEARS

Every unnecessary emergency room visit represents a missed opportunity for better care. Every avoided emergency room visit when care is truly needed represents a lost chance at life-saving intervention. Both patterns contribute to the decade of life that healthcare disparities are stealing from Black communities.

But when we learn to use the healthcare system strategically, emergency care for emergencies, urgent care for urgent issues, primary care for ongoing health management, we can improve outcomes while reducing costs and stress.

The emergency room will always be there when you truly need it. It shouldn't be your only option for healthcare, and it shouldn't be avoided when your life depends on it. Understanding the difference could add years to your life and life to your years.

Your health is too important to leave to emergency situations alone. Building a broader healthcare team, learning to recognize different types of health concerns, and knowing where to seek appropriate care are skills that can literally save your life.

The decade we're losing isn't just about delayed diagnoses or poor treatment of chronic diseases, it's also about using healthcare resources ineffectively and missing opportunities for prevention and early intervention. Learning to navigate the healthcare system more strategically is one more tool in the fight to reclaim those lost years.

Kid Comer's faith was strong, but it wasn't meant to replace medical care when she truly needed it. Similarly, the emergency room is a powerful resource when used appropriately, but it's not meant to replace all other forms of healthcare. Finding the balance between these extremes is part of becoming an informed healthcare consumer and protecting your most valuable asset: your health.

TIPS FROM DR. CARLA'S CARING CORNER

- Hire a professional clinician like a doctoral-prepared registered nurse to make intermittent visits to your church or business to educate your clients. The information they receive can extend their lives, where you get another decade to cut or style their hair.
- It is imperative that trusted places e.g. barbershops, beauty shops, and even churches enlist qualified healthcare people to address the health & wellness of parishioners. Though well-meaning, misinformation can be deadly to your customers.

- Partner with other community-based organizations (CBOs) to bring health & wellness events/activities to your business. Misinformation is as deadly as some diseases.
- If you work in the public sector, advise clients that you have developed close relationships with, resist the urge to offer any advice based on either your personal health experiences or that of other customers. Your medication and diseases are unique to you, not anyone else.
- If you are on the planning committee of a beauty or barber event, retain a doctoral-prepared registered nurse as a vendor in this space.

CHAPTER 7

The Power of Self-Advocacy – Taking Control of Your Health

The examination room can feel like foreign territory. You're sitting there in a paper gown with your backside vented while someone in a white coat speaks in medical jargon you don't understand. They're rushing, checking their watch, already mentally moving on to the next patient. You have questions, but you're not sure if you're allowed to ask them.

For Black patients, this scenario carries additional challenges. We're more likely to have our concerns dismissed or receive rushed explanations. But here's what you need to know: you have power in that room. You have the right to ask questions, demand clear explanations, and refuse treatments that don't make sense to you.

Learning to advocate for yourself transforms you from a passive patient into an active partner in your healthcare and that transformation can literally save your life.

WHEN SPEAKING UP CHANGES EVERYTHING

I once witnessed a situation involving a Black veteran in Mississippi who had been labeled a "frequent flier" in a local ER because he came in often complaining of pain. Over time, staff began to use bias-language like drug-seeking rather than suffering. His pain was dismissed. His visits were minimized.

During one visit, he made his way out of the emergency room and onto a medical unit. Staff became alarmed. Security gathered. The hallway was filled with people. Instantly, he was treated like a threat instead of a patient.

The chief nursing officer, a Black woman, was called to neutralize the situation. When she arrived, she declined a security escort. She went in alone, sat down nearest the exit, lowered her voice, and asked him to talk to her. He told her about his pain. He told her about how he was being treated. Then he showed her the scars from major shoulder surgeries he sustained after the war.

He was not drug-seeking. He was hurting. And he was not being heard.

She escorted him out safely and ensured that a physician would address his pain. She believed him, and because she did, his outcome changed completely.

WHEN OTHERS ADVOCATE FOR YOU

John was a Black man living in Washington, D.C. who had finally found love later in life. His wife noticed changes in him. He was moving slower, and napping more. She encouraged him to see a doctor, but he refused.

One day while she was at work, John's barber called to say her husband had slumped over in his barber chair and 911 had been called. His wife stayed with him during his hospitalization because she didn't trust the quality of care. She leaned on a close family friend who was a nurse to help translate what the doctors were saying.

After discharge, he continued to decline. She didn't accept vague answers from clinicians. She called around, found another doctor, and made the appointment herself. That's when they learned he had metastatic cancer.

Even as he remained in denial, she continued to fight for him. She attended every oncology appointment. She sought second opinions. She eventually left her job to care for him. She carried information he didn't want to hear and asked questions he wouldn't ask.

WHEN KNOWLEDGE BECOMES ACTION

Russ, a sixty-two-year-old Black man, complained to his wife of not feeling well. She noticed his decreased appetite and increased fatigue. His wife urged him multiple times to go to the hospital, but he repeatedly refused.

One day she found him in the bathroom vomiting lime green fluid. When she asked if he had, "eaten anything green?", he said, "no." She pleaded with him to allow her to call an ambulance, and still he disagreed.

His wife knew that lime green vomit was bile, a sign of a bowel obstruction, a serious condition requiring emergency surgery. She explained this to him, and finally he agreed to go to the emergency room, where he underwent immediate emergency surgery.

Her health knowledge literally saved his life.

OVERCOMING COMMON BARRIERS

Many people struggle with advocating for themselves in medical settings, but understanding these barriers is the first step to overcoming them. Fear and intimidation are common experiences, especially in medical settings that can feel overwhelming by design. The white coats, formal language, and institutional authority can make patients feel powerless. For Black patients who may have experienced discrimination, this intimidation is often magnified. The key is remembering that you have rights as a patient, regardless of how you're being treated.

Lack of medical knowledge often keeps people from asking questions because they're afraid of sounding uninformed. But here's the truth: it's the healthcare provider's job to explain things in ways you can understand. If you don't understand something, that's a failure of communication on their part, not a reflection of your intelligence.

Time constraints create another barrier when healthcare providers seem rushed, making patients feel they shouldn't ask questions or take up too much time. Your health is too important to sacrifice to someone else's schedule. Come prepared with your most important questions written down, and don't let yourself be rushed out until you get the information you need.

ESSENTIAL ADVOCACY TOOLS

One of the most powerful tools for patient advocacy is the "Ask Me 3: Good Questions for Your Good Health" framework developed by the Partnership for Clear Health Communication. These three simple questions can transform any medical encounter: What is my main problem? What do I need to do? Why is it important for me to do this? These questions ensure you leave every appointment understanding your diagnosis, treatment plan, and why it matters. They're simple enough to remember even when you're stressed and give you a framework for getting the most important information.

When you receive a diagnosis, you need to understand what you're dealing with. Ask your provider to explain the condition in simple terms, discuss how serious it is, what caused it, and what will happen if it's not treated. Don't accept vague explanations or medical jargon that leaves you confused.

For any recommended treatment, you deserve to know all your options. Ask about the benefits and risks of each approach, how long treatment will take, and what side effects you should expect. Understanding your alternatives helps you make informed decisions about your care.

When it comes to medications, knowledge can prevent dangerous mistakes and improve effectiveness. Make sure you understand what each medication is supposed to do, how and when to take it, what side effects to watch for, and whether there are any interactions with other drugs or foods you should know about.

PRACTICAL STRATEGIES FOR SUCCESS

Having someone with you during medical appointments can significantly improve your healthcare experience. A support person can take notes while you focus on listening, ask questions you might forget, provide emotional support, and serve as a witness to what was said. This is particularly important for complex diagnoses or treatment decisions where having a second set of ears can be invaluable.

Documentation is crucial for effective self-advocacy. Keep detailed records of all your appointments and what was discussed, your medications and any side effects you experience, questions you want to ask at future visits, and test results along with explanations of what they mean. This information helps you track patterns, remember important details, and provides evidence if you need to advocate with other providers or insurance companies.

Preparation before appointments makes advocacy much more effective. Write down your questions beforehand so you don't forget them in the moment. Bring a current list of all medications, including over-the-counter drugs and supplements. Know your family health history, and always bring your insurance cards and identification. This preparation shows providers you're engaged in your care and helps ensure you get the information you need.

DEALING WITH BIAS AND DISCRIMINATION

Unfortunately, bias in healthcare is real, and recognizing it is the first step to addressing it effectively. Bias might show up as rushed or dismissive communication, assumptions about your lifestyle or compliance with treatment, reluctance to provide adequate pain management or treatment options, or failure to take your concerns seriously. Knowing what to look for helps you respond appropriately.

When you encounter bias, staying calm but assertive is most effective. Ask for explanations in writing, request to speak with a supervisor if needed, and don't hesitate to seek second opinions. Document any discriminatory treatment carefully, including dates, names, and specific incidents. This documentation can be crucial if you need to file complaints, receive a custom satisfaction survey or seek care elsewhere.

BUILDING YOUR ADVOCACY SKILLS

If advocating for yourself feels overwhelming, start with small steps that build confidence over time. Ask one additional question at each appointment, request written instructions for anything you don't understand, and ask for copies of your test results. Each small action builds your comfort with speaking up and asking for what you need.

Practice these conversations at home with family members. Role-playing difficult scenarios helps you become more comfortable with advocacy language and builds confidence for real medical encounters. The more you practice, the more natural these interactions will feel.

Many communities have resources specifically designed to help patients become better advocates. Look for patient advocacy programs, community health workers, or patient navigator services in your area. These resources can provide training, support, and sometimes even accompaniment to important medical appointments.

YOUR VOICE MATTERS

Effective advocacy improves not just your own care but makes it easier for other Black patients who come after you. Every time you ask thoughtful questions, demand respectful treatment, and refuse to accept substandard care, you help change the culture of healthcare delivery.

The veteran in Mississippi needed someone who would listen and believe him. John needed someone who wouldn't accept his denial and would fight for his care. Russ needed someone who recognized the signs of a medical emergency and refused to take no for an answer.

Learning to advocate for yourself or having others advocate effectively for you, transforms passive healthcare experiences into active partnerships. Your questions matter, your concerns are valid, and your health is worth fighting for.

Those extra years that healthcare disparities threaten to steal from our communities can be reclaimed through effective advocacy, one conversation at a time. Each time you speak up, you're not just protecting your own health, you're helping to create a healthcare system that works better for everyone who looks like you.

TIPS FROM DR. CARLA'S CARING CORNER

- Advocates, like doctoral prepared Black nurses are trained professionals who know your struggles and teach you how to navigate the healthcare arena.
- Everyone is born with bias including healthcare workers. Recognizing implicit bias and bias language and implementing strategies to counter it is the way to extinguish it.
- Holding a visitors lounge hostage in a militant attempt to get attention is never the way. You may wind up a 5150 (temporary mental health hold), arrested for disturbing the peace, or killed while being subdued.
- Never lie about your narcotic use because ER doctors have the ability to look up said prescriptions on an app then your credibility is shot.
- Accept the offering of seeing a pain-management specialist when offered so you can have a better quality of life not dependent upon narcotic use.

- Narcotics don't just relieve pain. Simple pain relievers like Tylenol can constipate you and even be nephrotoxic (destroy your kidneys) making you a candidate for dialysis for life.

[Related to Second Story]

- Doctoral prepared nurses can help patients and family navigate the end-of-life process without feeling guilty, afraid, or overwhelmed.
- As soon as you become aware that your loved one has a terminal diagnosis, ask your doctor for a hospice referral. This does not signal you are rushing death but that you want to provide comfort, dignity and peace for this end-of-life journey.
- Death is nothing to be afraid of. It is only the living who can hurt you. It's ok to die at home.
- FYI, the law states when you are selling a home where there has been a death, it must be disclosed during the sale so looking for the small print. Disclosure is not a bad thing but it is the LAW. Just something to be considered.
- Black people can and should be open to hospice care. If not offered...inquire yourself before your loved one is discharged from the hospital.
- Just because you have a terminal illness and expected to die, you can still have hospice come to your home. You should not become a prisoner in your home just because you have been given a terminal diagnosis...so LIVE!

[From 3rd story]

- If you suspect a bowel obstruction, remain nothing per os (NPO) meaning don't eat or drink any more as you will probably go directly to surgery from the emergency room.
- Unless you know you have eaten something and can account for a particular color, assume there is something wrong if vomitus is colorful like lime green or yellow (bile), red (fresh bleeding), even black (old bleeding).
- Bile spilling out into the abdomen or stomach, not relieved, can begin to poison the patient internally setting up an infectious environment leading to possible severe illness or death.

CHAPTER 8

Bringing Health Education to Black Communities

Walk into any Black church on Sunday morning, and you'll hear conversations about everything from politics to family drama to who needs prayer for their health struggles. Sit in a barbershop on Saturday afternoon, and you'll witness debates about sports, current events, and inevitably, someone's medical situation that "the doctors can't figure out." Visit a community center during a health fair, and you'll see neighbors checking each other's blood pressure, sharing stories about medications, and trading advice about managing diabetes.

These spaces e.g., churches, barbershops, beauty salons, community centers have always been where Black communities gather information, share experiences, and look out for one another. They're also where health misinformation can spread just as quickly as accurate information, where old wives' tales mix with medical facts, and where historical mistrust of healthcare gets reinforced through shared stories.

But here's what's powerful about these spaces: they're also where real change can happen. When health education comes from trusted voices in familiar places, when it's delivered with cultural understanding and genuine care, these community spaces become powerful tools for extending lives and improving health outcomes.

The question isn't whether Black communities need health education, we clearly do, given the health disparities we face. The question is how to deliver that education in ways that people will trust, understand, and act upon.

WHEN COMMUNITY EDUCATION IS MISSING

The absence of culturally competent health education in Black communities has real consequences that play out in hospitals and homes across America every day. These aren't just statistics, they're stories of families who needed information that never reached them.

A nineteen-year-old Black woman married right out of high school to a blue-collar worker. He was employed by a reputable company specializing in manufacturing air compressors. She was a stay-at-home mom, and life was good. With her husband's excellent insurance, she was afforded quality prenatal care and went to all her scheduled doctor's appointments.

When she moved away from her family to marry, she had no one to provide the culturally competent prenatal information she needed. Even when she went for checkups, she never really knew what to ask or expect because this was her first child. What she did do frequently was board the South Shore train to visit her parents a few times a month. This train ride jostled her about in her pregnant state. No one ever told her that maybe this wasn't the best transportation choice for someone in the formative years of fetal development.

One Saturday, her husband dropped her off at the laundromat when suddenly she felt something wet and warm flow down her legs. She initially thought she had wet herself, but she had just used the bathroom moments earlier. She called her husband, who came and got her. While at home, she started experiencing severe abdominal pain and cramps, so they went to the hospital. Her baby wasn't due for another three months, so she knew enough to worry.

She spent hours in labor and delivery when they finally told her the baby was coming. She distinctly remembers lying on the delivery table when the obstetrician-gynecologist leaned down and whispered in her ear, "Your baby will probably be born dead." For a fleeting moment, she considered not participating in the delivery. Why push out a dead baby, she thought. She quietly prayed and started to push, delivering a baby girl.

It seemed like forever as they worked to get the baby to cry, but she finally did. Not a strong cry, but a cry nonetheless. The newborn wasn't out of the woods because she was born weighing 2 pounds, 4 ounces, less than a 5-pound bag of sugar from the grocery store. At that time, babies weren't allowed to leave the hospital until they weighed 5 pounds, so she was whisked away in her very first helicopter ride to a nearby hospital with a neonatal intensive care unit (NICU), where she spent her first 39 days of life. Mom was discharged but ordered to stay homebound for weeks. She never saw her baby in the NICU, that responsibility fell to her husband.

This could have been a story about maternal-infant mortality (death of mother and baby), as the majority of them are in our communities. Instead, it's a story of a high-risk pregnancy and how mother and baby fought to live despite a system that didn't educate her as extensively as it would have her white counterpart. Why wasn't anyone concerned with this young mother's frequent train rides? Why didn't anyone connect her with a doula from her community? Why wasn't she encouraged to provide breast-milk? Many Black babies die each year due to lack of education and information provided to parents, yet the system continues unchanged.

I lived to share this story.

WHEN COMMUNITY EDUCATION WORKS

Community-based health education can be transformative when it's done right. I've seen the power of meeting people where they are, with information they can trust, delivered by people who understand their lives.

Vonda, a 50 year old Black woman, attended a community event where she stopped at the table of a local Black Nurses Association offering free blood pressure checks. A doctoral-prepared registered nurse found her blood pressure to be dangerously high, almost 200mmHG for the top number (also called a systolic pressure).

She was advised to seek urgent care. The doctoral-prepared nurse took the time to educate her about what it means to have a systolic blood pressure that high. The nurse asked about her medication history when she blurted out, "Nurse, I'm just going to tell you the truth, I cannot afford the medication that was prescribed by my doctor."

Not willing to leave her without a solution, the nurse asked her to take out her cell phone, and she took out hers. The nurse proceeded to teach her how to locate her medications for cheaper prices using several pharmaceutical apps. The young lady became almost tearful as she shared that no one had ever shown her how to use these resources. The nurse proceeded to provide her with another equally valuable alternative for getting her blood pressure medications.

Pharmaceutical representatives all across this country, visit doctor's offices daily, wanting nothing more than the provider's signature. Once they get it, they return to their vehicles and bring back armfuls of medication samples for providers to distribute to patients in hopes of increasing prescription use. These medication samples cost the provider nothing and are meant to be distributed to patients who need them or when providers aren't sure how patients will tolerate a full prescription.

Most patients don't know how to ask for samples, and those that do, are ashamed to let the doctor know that they are not able to afford new prescriptions. It is ok to ask your doctor if he has any free samples available. During this encounter, the nurse noticed a small child with the young lady. When asked if the child was hers, she replied this was her grandchild and that her daughter had recently passed away and she was now raising her. Raising a school-age child, while on a fixed income, when you can't afford your blood pressure medications is a lost decade waiting to happen. Her daughter had already proven that.

That conversation at a community table lasted maybe fifteen minutes, but it potentially added years to Vonda's life. She learned about resources she didn't know existed, understood the seriousness of her condition, and felt heard and supported by someone who looked like her and understood her struggles.

THE UNIQUE POWER OF COMMUNITY SPACES

Black communities have always turned to trusted spaces for information and support, and these spaces offer unique advantages for health education that formal healthcare settings often can't match.

Churches reach people who might never set foot in a doctor's office until they're having a medical emergency. When health information comes from the pulpit or through health ministry programs, it carries the weight of spiritual authority and community trust. Pastor-led health initiatives have successfully addressed everything from diabetes management to mental health awareness because they frame health as stewardship of the body God gave us.

Barbershops and beauty salons create natural opportunities for health conversations in relaxed, familiar environments. When the person cutting your hair mentions their experience managing high blood pressure, that information carries different weight than the same advice from a rushed doctor. These spaces also reach men who are notoriously difficult to engage in health education through traditional channels.

Community centers, health fairs, and local events provide opportunities for hands-on education and immediate action. People can get screenings, ask questions, and receive resources all in one place. When these events are organized by trusted community organizations, they feel safe and welcoming rather than clinical and intimidating.

OVERCOMING HISTORICAL BARRIERS

Bringing effective health education to Black communities requires understanding and addressing the barriers that have made previous efforts unsuccessful. The historical mistrust we've discussed throughout this book doesn't disappear just because someone has good intentions and helpful information.

Cultural factors play a huge role in how health messages are received. Information that contradicts deeply held beliefs about faith, family roles, or traditional remedies needs to be presented carefully and respectfully. Effective community health education doesn't dismiss these beliefs but rather works to integrate accurate medical information with cultural values and practices.

Language and communication style matter enormously. Medical jargon doesn't work in community settings, but neither does talking down to people or oversimplifying complex issues. The most effective community health educators are those who can translate medical information into everyday language while respecting people's intelligence and life experience.

Trust must be earned rather than assumed. Communities that have been exploited by researchers, abandoned by healthcare systems, or ignored by public health initiatives have learned to be skeptical of outside health messages. Successful community health education often starts with listening, understanding what the community already knows, what their concerns are, and what they most need to learn.

THE ROLE OF TRUSTED LEADERS

Community leaders who are effective health educators share certain qualities that make their messages more likely to be heard and acted upon. They have established credibility within the community through years of service and authentic relationships. They understand the cultural context and can frame health information in ways that resonate with community values. They're accessible and approachable rather than distant or authoritarian.

The most effective community health educators often aren't healthcare professionals at all. They're pastors who integrate health messages into spiritual teachings, barbers who share their own health journeys while cutting hair, and community mothers who look out for their neighbors' wellbeing. These individuals succeed because they're trusted messengers delivering important information in the context of existing relationships.

Healthcare professionals can be effective community educators when they approach communities as partners rather than experts coming to fix problems. The most successful medical professionals in community health education are those who listen first, respect community wisdom, and work collaboratively to address health concerns.

DIGITAL PLATFORMS AND MODERN CHALLENGES

Social media and digital platforms have created both opportunities and challenges for community health education. On one hand, these platforms can rapidly spread accurate health information to large audiences, connect people with similar health conditions, and provide access to resources that might not be available locally.

On the other hand, these same platforms can spread health misinformation just as quickly, create echo chambers that reinforce dangerous beliefs, and provide platforms for conspiracy theories that prey on legitimate historical concerns. The challenge is helping communities navigate these digital spaces more effectively.

Successful digital health education in Black communities often comes from trusted voices who have built authentic online followings. These might be healthcare professionals who create content specifically for Black audiences, community advocates who share their own health journeys, or organizations that consistently provide reliable health information.

The key is teaching people to evaluate online health information critically. This includes checking sources, looking for medical credentials, being skeptical of miracle cures, and consulting healthcare professionals before making major health decisions based on social media content.

Critical evaluation is just the beginning. As our communities become increasingly connected through smartphones, tablets, and social media, we need to develop specific digital health literacy skills such as the ability to find, understand, and use online health information effectively. These skills are becoming just as important as traditional health literacy, and when mastered, they can be powerful tools for closing the health gap that has persisted in our communities for far too long.

STRATEGIES THAT WORK

The most effective community health education initiatives share several common elements that make them successful in reaching and influencing Black communities.

They start with community assessment and engagement, taking time to understand what health issues the community prioritizes, what barriers they face in accessing care, and what communication methods are most likely to be effective. This groundwork ensures that programs address real needs rather than imposed priorities.

Successful programs use multiple touchpoints and reinforcement strategies. A single health fair or workshop rarely changes behavior, but ongoing programs that provide repeated exposure to health messages through various channels can create lasting change. This might include combining church-based education with barbershop conversations, social media campaigns, and peer support groups.

Investing in quality expertise is essential for effective community health education. Too often, churches, community centers, and other organizations expect healthcare providers like doctors, doctoral-prepared nurses, nurse practitioners, and specialists to donate their time and expertise without compensation. While the intention is good, this approach can actually limit access to the best information our communities need.

Healthcare providers have invested years of their lives and hundreds of thousands of dollars in their education and training. When we consistently expect them to share this expertise for free, we create several problems: we limit which providers are willing to participate, we may get rushed or superficial information rather than thorough education, and we undervalue the very knowledge that could save lives in our communities.

The most successful community health programs recognize that quality health education is worth paying for. They build compensation into their budgets, seek grants that include provider fees, or find creative ways to fairly compensate health professionals for their time and expertise. This investment attracts better providers, ensures more comprehensive information, and creates sustainable programs that can continue long-term.

When Vonda received life-saving information about her blood pressure and medication resources, it was because a doctoral-prepared nurse was being properly compensated for her time at that community event. That compensation allowed the nurse to sit with her, provide thorough education, and ensure she had the resources she needed. Free or underpaid expertise often means rushed interactions that miss these crucial details.

Cultural competence is essential but goes beyond surface-level accommodations. Truly culturally competent health education understands the historical context, addresses specific concerns that Black communities face, and respects the wisdom and strength that these communities possess.

Partnership and sustainability ensure that programs continue beyond initial funding or enthusiasm. The most successful community health education initiatives are those that build local capacity, train community members to continue the work, and integrate health education into existing community structures.

CREATING LASTING CHANGE

Effective community health education doesn't just inform people, it empowers them to make different choices, advocate for better care, and share accurate information with others. When Vonda learned about medication assistance programs at that community event, she didn't just benefit herself, she became someone who could share that knowledge with other community members facing similar challenges.

When expectant mothers receive culturally competent prenatal education, they're better equipped to advocate for themselves and their babies, potentially preventing complications and improving outcomes. When barbershops become spaces for honest conversations about men's health, they can reach men who might otherwise avoid health care entirely.

These ripple effects are how community-based health education can help reclaim some of those lost years that health disparities have stolen from Black communities. Each person who receives accurate, culturally relevant health information becomes a potential educator for others. Each successful intervention creates models that can be replicated in other communities.

The power to improve health outcomes in Black communities doesn't just rest with nurses, doctors, hospitals, and healthcare systems. It also lies within our own communities, in our churches, barbershops, community centers, and social networks. When we harness that power effectively, when we combine community wisdom with medical knowledge, when we create space for honest conversations about health in trusted environments, we can begin to address the health disparities that have persisted for far too long.

Your community has the power to extend lives, improve health outcomes, and fight back against the misinformation that costs us years of life. The question is how we'll choose to use that power and whether we'll commit to making health education a community priority that reaches everyone who needs it.

TIPS FROM DR. CARLA'S CARING CORNER

- Black Doula's have been shown to increase the birthing experience for mother/baby. Find a doula in your area or ask your family and friends at church and in the community if they know someone.
- Doula's do not have to be nurses or someone you know. They are trained to support you through your pregnancy.
- Any time you can spend breastfeeding your baby is an opportunity to help him develop and grow strong. Request the labor and delivery nurse send the la leche nurse to see you for breastfeeding training/education before going home.

- Tell your doctor or other members of the healthcare team about your experiences e.g. what type of work you do, how often or long is your commute, when should you stop flying or using stairs, if you are addicted to prescription or illegal drugs, are experiencing domestic violence or human trafficking to name a few. Assume nothing and share everything so that you deliver a healthy baby.

- Prenatal visits and prescribed prenatal vitamins can save you and your baby's life.

[From second story]

- Downloadable prescription Apps e.g. Good Rx and Singlecare where you can enter a few pieces of information e.g. medication name, dose like how many milligrams, and quantity like the number of pills e.g., 30, 60 or 90 day supply and get results of multiple nearby pharmacies who charge almost pennies for most prescriptions.

- Not all pharmacies prioritize whether you can afford your medication. When you walk up to the counter, pull up your app e.g. Singlecare or GoodRx and see if the price is cheaper. Remember, they are not in business to save you money so have this app pulled up when you step up to the counter.

- It is ok to say to the pharmacists, "is this the cheapest that I can get this prescription here?" You would be surprised at the answer.

- Ask the prescribing physician if there are any samples of this prescription that you can get from him today. This may buy you some time and certainly save you some money.

CHAPTER 9

Digital Health Literacy – Using Technology to Close the Gap

Your smartphone is more powerful than the computers that sent humans to the moon, yet when it comes to managing your health, you might feel like you're still in the Stone Age. You can order food, manage your finances, and video chat with family across the country with a few taps, but finding reliable health information online feels overwhelming and confusing.

This digital divide in healthcare isn't just about convenience, it's about life and death. In an age where telemedicine appointments can prevent emergency room visits, where apps can help manage chronic diseases, and where reliable health information is available 24/7, being digitally disconnected means being healthcare disconnected.

But here's the challenge: the same technology that can extend your life can also endanger it. The internet that provides access to world-class medical information also spreads dangerous health myths at lightning speed. The social media platforms that connect you with supportive communities also amplify voices that profit from your confusion and fear.

Learning to navigate digital health resources effectively isn't just about keeping up with technology, it's about taking control of your health in an increasingly digital world. It's about distinguishing between life-saving information and life-threatening misinformation. It's about using technology to reclaim some of those lost years that healthcare disparities have stolen from our communities.

THE PROMISE OF DIGITAL HEALTH TOOLS

Digital health technology has the potential to revolutionize healthcare for Black communities in ways that could dramatically reduce health disparities. When used effectively, these tools can provide access to care that geography, economics, and systemic barriers have traditionally denied us.

Telehealth services can connect you with healthcare providers without the barriers of transportation, time off work, or childcare challenges. During the COVID-19 pandemic, many people discovered they could have meaningful conversations with their doctors from their living rooms, asking questions they might have felt rushed to ask in person, getting medication adjustments without missing work, and receiving follow-up care that might otherwise have been skipped.

Health monitoring apps can help you track blood pressure, blood sugar, medication adherence, and symptoms in ways that provide both you and your healthcare providers with detailed information about your health patterns. Instead of trying to remember how you felt over the past three months during a brief doctor's appointment, you can show real data about your daily experiences.

Educational platforms and reliable health websites can provide culturally relevant health information that addresses the specific concerns and conditions that disproportionately affect Black communities. You can learn about managing diabetes, understanding heart disease risk factors, or preparing for medical procedures at your own pace, in your own space, without feeling judged or rushed.

Medication management tools can send reminders, track side effects, identify potential interactions, and even help you find affordable alternatives or assistance programs. These tools can turn medication management from a source of confusion and stress into a manageable part of daily life.

THE DIGITAL DIVIDE IN HEALTHCARE

Accessing these digital health benefits requires overcoming significant barriers that disproportionately affect Black communities. The same systemic inequities that create healthcare disparities also create digital health disparities.

Internet access remains inconsistent in many Black communities, with slower speeds, higher costs, and less reliable service than in affluent areas. When telehealth appointments require high-speed internet for video calls, when health apps need constant connectivity to sync data, and when online resources require significant bandwidth to load properly, unreliable internet becomes a health equity issue.

Digital literacy varies widely within communities, and healthcare technology often assumes a level of technical comfort that not everyone possesses. Older adults who didn't grow up with smartphones, people who use technology primarily for basic communication, and those who've had limited exposure to health apps may find these tools more frustrating than helpful without proper support and training.

Device access creates another layer of inequality. While smartphones are common, not everyone has devices capable of running complex health apps, supporting video calls, or storing large amounts of health data. Older phones with limited memory and processing power can't take advantage of many digital health innovations.

Cost considerations affect everything from data plans to app subscriptions to device upgrades. When families are choosing between paying for high-speed internet and other necessities, digital health tools become luxuries rather than essential healthcare resources.

THE MISINFORMATION CRISIS

The same digital platforms that can provide life-saving health information also serve as superhighways for dangerous misinformation. Social media algorithms that prioritize engagement often amplify sensational health claims over boring but accurate medical facts. Conspiracy theories that prey on legitimate historical concerns about medical racism can spread faster than scientific evidence that could save lives.

Health misinformation in Black communities often exploits real experiences of discrimination and medical neglect. When someone shares a story about poor treatment in a hospital, it resonates with people who've had similar experiences. When that story gets mixed with false claims about medications or vaccines, the legitimate grievance provides credibility to dangerous misinformation.

The speed and scale of digital misinformation make it particularly dangerous. A false claim about diabetes medication or blood pressure treatment can reach thousands of people in hours, potentially causing them to stop taking life-saving medications or avoid necessary medical care. Unlike misinformation spread through conversation, digital misinformation can appear more credible with fake testimonials, doctored images, and links to websites designed to look legitimate.

Economic incentives fuel much health misinformation. People selling supplements, alternative treatments, or conspiracy theories profit when others distrust conventional medicine. They use sophisticated digital marketing techniques to target vulnerable communities with messages designed to exploit fears and promote distrust.

BUILDING DIGITAL HEALTH LITERACY SKILLS

Developing digital health literacy requires learning to evaluate online health information critically while taking advantage of legitimate digital health resources. These skills are becoming as important as traditional health literacy for navigating modern healthcare effectively.

Learning to identify credible sources is fundamental to digital health literacy. Reliable health websites typically end in .gov, .edu, or .org, are affiliated with established medical institutions, cite scientific research, and are written or reviewed by healthcare professionals with clear credentials. They present balanced information about benefits and risks rather than promising miracle cures or demonizing conventional treatments.

Understanding how to fact-check health claims can protect you from dangerous misinformation. This means looking for multiple reliable sources that support the same conclusions, checking publication dates to ensure information is current, and being skeptical of dramatic claims that seem too good to be true or that contradict established medical knowledge.

Recognizing red flags in health information helps you avoid dangerous advice. Be suspicious of sources that discourage you from consulting healthcare professionals, promise quick fixes for complex health problems, use dramatic testimonials instead of scientific evidence, or try to sell you specific products while providing health advice.

Learning to use telehealth effectively maximizes the benefits of digital healthcare access. This includes having good lighting and minimal background noise for video calls, preparing questions in advance, having medications and health information readily available, and understanding how to use the technology before your appointment starts.

THE ROLE OF HEALTHCARE PROVIDERS IN DIGITAL HEALTH

Healthcare providers and community leaders play crucial roles in helping patients navigate digital health resources safely and effectively. They serve as filters, guides, and educators who can help distinguish between helpful technology and dangerous misinformation.

Doctors and nurses who recommend specific health apps, websites, or digital tools provide valuable guidance that can save patients hours of searching and protect them from unreliable sources. When healthcare providers integrate digital tools into care plans, they can monitor how patients use these resources and provide feedback about their effectiveness.

Community health workers and patient navigators can provide hands-on training in digital health literacy, helping people learn to use telehealth platforms, health monitoring apps, and reliable health websites. This type of practical education addresses both technical skills and critical evaluation abilities.

Faith leaders, barbers, and other trusted community voices can promote digital health literacy by modeling good information-seeking behavior, sharing reliable sources when health topics arise in conversation, and encouraging people to fact-check health information before acting on it or sharing it with others.

Healthcare institutions can improve digital health equity by providing device lending programs, offering technical support for telehealth appointments, creating multilingual digital health resources, and ensuring their own digital platforms are accessible to users with varying levels of digital literacy.

MAKING DIGITAL HEALTH INCLUSIVE

Creating digital health solutions that truly serve Black communities requires intentional design that addresses the specific barriers and needs these communities face. This goes beyond simply making existing tools available to everyone, it requires building equity into the technology itself.

Culturally relevant content makes digital health tools more effective for Black users. This means featuring diverse representation in images and videos, addressing health conditions that disproportionately affect Black communities, acknowledging historical medical context when appropriate, and using language and examples that resonate with Black cultural experiences.

Accessibility features ensure that digital health tools work for users with different abilities, internet speeds, and device capabilities. This includes designing apps that function on older smartphones, creating content that loads quickly on slower internet connections, offering text-based alternatives to video content, and providing multiple ways to access the same information.

Affordability considerations make digital health tools realistic options for people with limited economic resources. This might involve offering free versions of health apps, partnering with community organizations to provide device access, working with internet service providers to offer reduced-cost plans for health purposes, or integrating digital health tools into existing community health programs.

Community partnerships help ensure that digital health innovations actually reach and benefit the communities they're designed to serve. This means working with trusted local organizations, incorporating community feedback into design processes, providing ongoing technical support and training, and measuring success based on community-defined outcomes rather than just technology adoption rates.

THE FUTURE OF HEALTH EQUITY

Digital health technology will continue to evolve, creating new opportunities and challenges for healthcare equity. Artificial intelligence could provide personalized health guidance, but only if it's trained on diverse data that includes Black experiences. Virtual reality might revolutionize health education, but only if it's accessible to communities that need it most. Wearable devices could provide continuous health monitoring, but only if they work accurately on dark skin and are affordable for everyone.

The key is ensuring that Black communities are not just consumers of digital health technology but active participants in its development and implementation. This means having Black voices in technology companies, healthcare institutions, and policy-making processes that determine how digital health evolves.

It also means continuing to build digital health literacy skills within our communities so that we can take advantage of beneficial innovations while protecting ourselves from harmful ones. The same critical thinking skills that help you evaluate health information online can help you assess new health technologies as they emerge.

RECLAIMING TIME THROUGH TECHNOLOGY

When used wisely, digital health technology can help reclaim some of those lost years that healthcare disparities have stolen from Black communities. Telehealth can provide earlier intervention for chronic diseases. Health monitoring apps can catch problems before they become emergencies. Reliable online health information can empower better decision-making and more effective self-advocacy.

This potential is realized only when digital health resources are accessible, trustworthy, and designed with equity in mind. It requires developing the skills to navigate digital health information safely and effectively. It requires healthcare providers and community leaders who actively support digital health literacy. It requires technology companies and healthcare institutions that prioritize equity in their digital health innovations.

Your smartphone and internet connection can be powerful tools for extending your life and improving your health if you know how to use them effectively. Learning digital health literacy skills isn't just about keeping up with technology; it's about using technology to take control of your health in ways that previous generations could never imagine.

The choice is yours: will you let digital health disparities widen the gap in health outcomes, or will you develop the skills needed to use technology as a tool for health equity? The future of healthcare is increasingly digital, and your ability to navigate that future effectively could determine how many healthy years you have ahead of you.

CHAPTER 10

Conclusion – Reclaiming Our Decade

Mary is still my aunt.

She still tells the same stories. She still recognizes people others forget. She still carries the history of her family in ways no record ever could. What nearly disappeared were the years she was meant to live those moments.

Mary did not lose a decade because she failed to care about her health. She did not lose it because she avoided doctors, ignored advice, or lacked discipline. She lost it because warning signs were treated as isolated problems, confusion was mistaken for understanding, and no one slowed the process down long enough to see the full picture.

What saved her was intervention.

Not perfection.

Not expertise.

Intervention.

Someone noticed patterns instead of symptoms. Someone questioned delays that felt routine. Someone refused to accept that showing up was enough when the outcome clearly was not improving.

Mary lived because someone stood in the gap.

Most people never get that moment.

That is the quiet truth behind the lost decade. Time is not usually stolen by one catastrophic event. It is lost inch by inch through misunderstandings, delayed follow-ups, unmanaged conditions, and systems that move forward whether clarity exists or not.

This book has shown you how that happens.

You have seen how limited healthcare literacy leaves patients nodding instead of knowing. How history shapes mistrust long before a patient ever enters an exam room. How structural barriers slow care until early becomes late. How preventable conditions turn deadly when no one intervenes early enough. How emergency care replaces continuity. How technology can either empower or overwhelm.

What matters now is what you do with that knowledge.

You do not need credentials to protect your health.

You do not need authority to ask questions.

You do not need permission to pause the process.

You can be Carla for yourself.

That looks like insisting on understanding before agreeing to a plan. It looks like asking what happens next, what should change, and what should never be ignored. It looks like recognizing when something feels off and refusing to minimize it. It looks like treating your health as something that requires engagement, not blind trust.

You can also be Carla for someone else.

For the parent who says they are fine but is slowly withdrawing.

For the relative whose condition keeps changing but never improving.

For the loved one who keeps ending up in the emergency room with no long-term plan.

Advocacy is not confrontation. It is presence. It is paying attention when systems move too fast. It is asking the questions others assume have already been answered.

This book was never meant to turn patients into clinicians or families into experts. It was meant to restore agency. To make sure that information leads to understanding, and understanding leads to action.

The lost decade is not inevitable.

It is not fate.

It is not just a statistic.

It is the result of silence, delay, and confusion.

Which means it can be interrupted.

The years ahead of you are not automatic. They will either be lived intentionally or quietly slip away through moments that feel insignificant at the time.

Mary almost lost ten years.

She did not because someone stepped in.

Now you know how to step in.

For yourself.

For others.

For the generations watching what you tolerate and what you challenge.

The decade is not gone yet.

It is still within reach.

Choose to live it.

REFERENCES

Caraballo, C., Massey, D. S., Ndumele, C. D., Haywood, T., Kaleem, S., King, T., Liu, Y., Lu, Y., Nunez-Smith, M., Taylor, H. A., Watson, K. E., Herrin, J., Yancy, C. W., Faust, J. S., & Krumholz, H. M. (2023). Excess mortality and years of potential life lost among the Black population in the US, 1999–2020. *JAMA*, 329(19), 1662–1670. https://doi.org/10.1001/jama.2023.7022

Centers for Disease Control and Prevention. (n.d.). *Health literacy*. https://www.cdc.gov/healthliteracy/learn/index.html

Centers for Disease Control and Prevention. (2024, October 16). *What is health literacy?* https://www.cdc.gov/health-literacy/php/about/index.html

Gunja, M. Z., Gumas, E. D., & Williams, R. D., II. (2023, January 31). U.S. health care from a global perspective, 2022: Accelerating spending, worsening outcomes. *The Commonwealth Fund*. https://www.commonwealthfund.

org/publications/issue-briefs/2023/jan/us-health-care-global-perspective-2022

Hall, G. L., & Heath, M. (2021). Poor medication adherence in African Americans is a matter of trust. *Journal of Racial and Ethnic Health Disparities*, *8*(4), 927–942. https://doi.org/10.1007/s40615-020-00850-3

Hughes-Halbert, C., Melvin, C., Briggs, V., Delmoor, E., Rice, L. J., Lynch, C., Jefferson, M., & Johnson, J. C. (2016). Neighborhood satisfaction and colorectal cancer screening in a community sample of African Americans. *Journal of Community Health*, *41*(1), 38–45. https://doi.org/10.1007/s10900-015-0062-9

Liu, C., Wang, D., Liu, C., Jiang, J., Wang, X., Chen, H., Ju, X., & Zhang, X. (2020). What is the meaning of health literacy? A systematic review and qualitative synthesis. *Family Medicine and Community Health*, *8*(2), e000351. https://doi.org/10.1136/fmch-2020-000351

Muvuka, B., Combs, R. M., Ayangeakaa, S. D., Ali, N. M., Wendel, M. L., & Jackson, T. (2020). Health literacy in African-American communities: Barriers and strategies. *HLRP: Health Literacy Research and Practice*, *4*(3), e138–e143. https://doi.org/10.3928/24748307-20200617-01

National Center for Education Statistics. (n.d.). *Health literacy component of the National Assessment of Adult Literacy (NAAL)*. U.S. Department of Education. https://nces.ed.gov/naal/health.asp

Office of Disease Prevention and Health Promotion. (n.d.). *Health literacy in Healthy People 2030*. U.S. Department of Health and Human Services. https://health.gov/our-work/national-health-initiatives/health-literacy

Office of Disease Prevention and Health Promotion. (n.d.). *Health literacy resources*. U.S. Department of Health and Human Services. https://odphp.health.gov/our-work/national-health-initiatives/health-literacy/resources

Perrenoud, B., Velonaki, V.-S., Bodenmann, P., & Ramelet, A.-S. (2015). The effectiveness of health literacy interventions on the informed consent process of health care users: A systematic review protocol. *JBI Database of Systematic Reviews and Implementation Reports*, *13*(10), 82–94. https://doi.org/10.11124/jbisrir-2015-2304

Rowlands, G., Shaw, A., Jaswal, S., Smith, S., & Harpham, T. (2017). Health literacy and the social determinants of health: A qualitative model from adult learners. *Health Promotion International*, *32*(1), 130–138. https://doi.org/10.1093/heapro/dav093

Santana, S., Brach, C., Harris, L., Ochiai, E., Blakey, C., Bevington, F., Kleinman, D., & Pronk, N. (2021). Updating health literacy for Healthy People 2030: Defining its importance for a new decade in public health. *Journal of Public Health Management and Practice*, *27*(Suppl. 6), S258–S264. https://doi.org/10.1097/PHH.0000000000001324

Sterling, E. W., Stevens, L., Robinson-Dooley, V., & Collette, T. (2025). Black men and health literacy: Strategies for improvement in a digital age through the adaptation of a chronic disease self-management program. *International Journal of Environmental Research and Public Health*, *22*(7), 1153. https://doi.org/10.3390/ijerph22071153

Turkson-Ocran, R.-A. N., Ogungbe, O., Botchway, M., Baptiste, D. L., Owusu, B., Ajibewa, T., Chen, Y., Gbaba,

S., Kwapong, F. L., Aidoo, E. L., Nmezi, N. A., Cluett, J. L., Commodore-Mensah, Y., & Juraschek, S. P. (2024). Hypertension management to reduce racial/ethnic disparities: Clinical and community-based interventions. *Current Cardiovascular Risk Reports, 18*(12), 239–258. https://doi.org/10.1007/s12170-024-00750-9

U.S. Bureau of Justice Statistics. (2025, September 30). *Prisoners in 2023 – Statistical tables*. U.S. Department of Justice. https://bjs.ojp.gov/library/publications/prisoners-2023-statistical-tables

U.S. Department of Health and Human Services, Office of Minority Health. (n.d.). *Infant mortality and Black/African Americans*. https://minorityhealth.hhs.gov/infant-health-and-mortality-and-blackafrican-americans

U.S. Department of Health and Human Services. (n.d.). *Health literacy reports and publications*. https://www.hhs.gov/surgeongeneral/reports-and-publications/health-literacy/

ACKNOWLEDGMENTS

No work like this is ever created alone, and I am deeply grateful for the people whose love, support, wisdom, and presence helped carry it into the world.

First, to my beloved husband, Russell, my partner of forty-six years: thank you for your unwavering support, your patience, and your quiet strength. You made room for this work in countless seen and unseen ways, and without you, this book would not have been possible.

To my daughter, Brandhyze, and my grandson, Samuel Jr., thank you for the joy you bring to my life. Your laughter, your love, and even the simple gift of our FaceTime moments sustained me more than you know.

To my mother, Mrs. Andrews, thank you for the discipline, faith, and character you poured into our family. The values you instilled continue to shape not only who I am, but also the message I hope this book carries forward.

I am also forever grateful for the legacy of those whose love, lessons, and example remain with me: Edward "Lil Bro" Riley,

John L. Andrews, King John L. Andrews, Tonia Jones, George and Clotee Thomas, Willie Davis, Queen, John and Maggie "Big Ma." Each of you has left an imprint on my life that lives within these pages.

A special thank-you to Geo Derice for the insight, thoughtful dialogue, and nuggets that helped shape direction of this book.

And to the family, friends, colleagues, and every person who shared their stories, wisdom, encouragement, and support along the way: thank you. This book may carry my name, but it has been shaped by the presence of many.

With humility and deep gratitude.

ABOUT THE AUTHOR

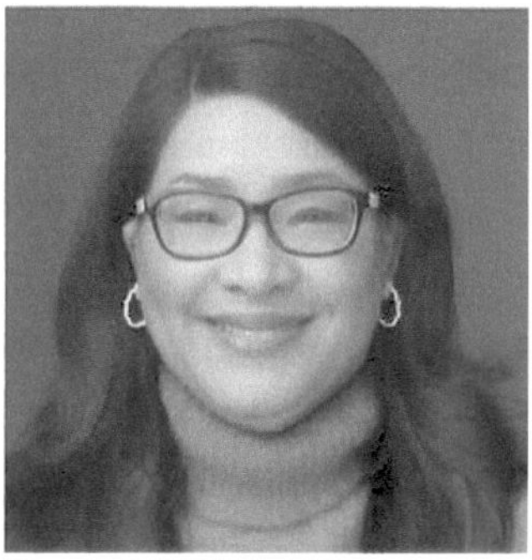

DR. CARLA STANLEY is a respected nurse leader, mentor, and advocate with more than thirty years of experience in acute critical care and healthcare leadership. A 2022 CAHL Service Award honoree, she is known for her commitment to service and her belief in helping others reach their goals. Raised by a pastor father who started his church in their family kitchen, Carla learned early what servant leadership looks like. She carries that spirit into every role, often saying she is driven to help people get to where they are trying to go.

A lifetime member of the National Black Nurses Association and past president of the Central Valley Black Nurses Association, Carla is deeply committed to advancing Black nurses and improving the health of BIPOC communities. Her career includes roles from bedside nurse to senior vice president, chief nursing officer, and now chief nurse executive for California Corrections Health Care Services, with clinical experience across seven states.

As a 2022 to 2023 American Nurses Association Fellow for Advocacy and Policy, she supports efforts to address Racism in Nursing and believes nurses must have a voice where decisions are made. Her motto is clear. If you are not at the table, you are on the menu.

Carla is currently pursuing her PhD at UCSF to stay relevant in her field and to inspire nurses of color. If you can see me, you can be me is the message she hopes to pass on. She continues to learn, grow, and lift others through mentorship, resources, and opportunities.

Her leadership values show up in stories like her CAHL moment, where one invitation sparked new relationships and inspired others to get involved. To Carla, that kind of warm, inclusive community is what leadership should create.

Carla is also a multi-board-certified expert, a sought-after panelist, and a strong voice for equitable care delivery across all communities. She lives by guiding principles that reflect her purpose. Evil prevails when good people do nothing. It is ok to fall if you fall forward. What would you do if you were not afraid. If not now, when. If not you, then who.

THE CONVERSATION DOES NOT HAVE TO END HERE

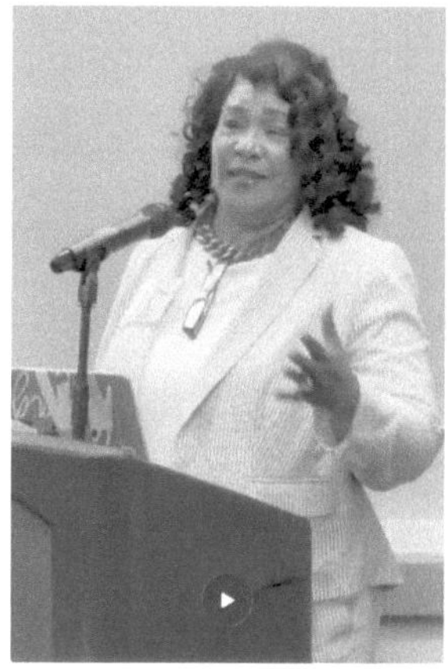

Throughout these pages, you have read about the power of having someone in your corner who knows the healthcare, knows the community, and knows how to translate one for the other in a way that saves lives.

That is not a hypothetical. That is what I do.

This book is the beginning. The gap starts closing when we get in the room together, make space for real conversation, and go deeper than any chapter can take you.

Some communities need someone to walk through the door, sit with the people, answer the hard questions, and make sure nobody leaves still in the dark. If that is your community, I am ready.

To inquire, email: **booking@vitalpathconsultingandeducation.com**

www.ingramcontent.com/pod-product-compliance
Ingram Content Group UK Ltd.
Pitfield, Milton Keynes, MK11 3LW, UK
UKHW041855031026
15587UKWH00007B/1238/J

9 798994 766705